Restless Legs Syndrome

Restless Legs Syndrome

Edited by

K. Ray Chaudhuri MD FRCP
The Movement Disorders Unit
King's College Hospital, and
University Hospital Lewisham
London, UK

P. Odin MD PhD
Department of Neurology
Zentralkrankenhaus Reinkenheide
Bremerhaven
Germany

C. W. Olanow MD
Department of Neurology
Mount Sinai Medical Center
New York, USA

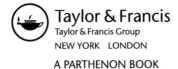

Taylor & Francis
Taylor & Francis Group
NEW YORK   LONDON

A PARTHENON BOOK

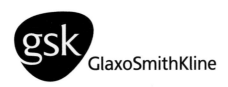

GlaxoSmithKline

© 2004 Taylor & Francis, an imprint of the Taylor & Francis Group

First published in the United Kingdom in 2004
by Taylor & Francis,
an imprint of the Taylor & Francis Group,
2 Park Square, Milton Park
Abingdon, Oxon OX14 4RN, UK

Tel.: +44 (0) 1235 828600
Fax.: +44 (0) 1235 829000
Website: www.tandf.co.uk

British Library Cataloguing in Publication Data

Data available on application

Library of Congress Cataloging-in-Publication Data

Data available on application

ISBN 1-84214-162-7

Distributed in North and South America by

Taylor & Francis
2000 NW Corporate Blvd
Boca Raton, FL 33431, USA

Within Continental USA
Tel.: 800 272 7737; Fax.: 800 374 3401
Outside Continental USA
Tel.: 561 994 0555; Fax.: 561 361 6018
E-mail: orders@crcpress.com

Distributed in the rest of the world by
Thomson Publishing Services
Cheriton House
North Way
Andover, Hampshire SP10 5BE, UK
Tel.: +44 (0) 1264 332424
E-mail: salesorder.tandf@thomsonpublishingservices.co.uk

Composition by Parthenon Publishing
Printed and bound by Antony Rowe Ltd., Chippenham, Wiltshire, UK

Contents

List of contributors

Dr K. Ray Chaudhuri
Department of Neurology
King's College Hospital
Denmark Hill
London SE5 9RS
UK

Dr Vandana Dhawan
University Hospital Lewisham
 and St. Thomas' Hospital
London SE5 9RS
UK

Dr Renata Egatz
Sleep Disorders Unit
Department of Neurology
Fundación Jiménez Díaz
Avda. Reyes Católicos 2
28040 Madrid
Spain

Dr Diego Garcia-Borreguero
Sleep Disorders Unit
Department of Neurology
Fundación Jiménez Díaz
Avda. Reyes Católicos 2
28040 Madrid
Spain

Dr Michael Jöbges
Neurological Rehabilitation Center
 Leipzig
Muldentalweg 1
04828 Bennewitz
Germany

Dr William Koller
Department of Neurology
Mount Sinai Medical Center
One Gustave L. Levy Place
New York, NY 10029
USA

Catherine Meilak
Guy's, King's, St.Thomas' School
 of Medicine
and King's College
London SE5 9RS
UK

Dr Matthias Mrowka
Department of Neurology
Zentralkrankenhaus Reinkenheide
Postbrockstrasse 103
27574 Bremerhaven
Germany

Professor Per Odin
Department of Neurology
Zentralkrankenhaus Reinkenheide
Postbrockstrasse 103
27574 Bremerhaven
Germany

Professor C. Warren Olanow
Department of Neurology
Mount Sinai Medical Center
One Gustave L. Levy Place
New York, NY 10029
USA

Dr William Ondo
Department of Neurology
Baylor College of Medicine
6550 Fannin, Suite 1801
Houston, TX 77030
USA

Dr Carolina Serrano
Sleep Disorders Unit
Department of Neurology
Fundación Jiménez Díaz
Avda. Reyes Católicos 2
28040 Madrid
Spain

Dr Winona Tse
Department of Neurology
Mount Sinai Medical Center
One Gustave L. Levy Place
New York, NY 10029
USA

Preface

Restless legs syndrome (RLS) is the commonest movement disorder, affecting as many as 10% of individuals. Nonetheless, its cause is unknown. Only a small percentage of patients who suffer from this disorder are accurately diagnosed, and the frequency with which patients suffer clinical disability as a consequence of RLS is not fully appreciated. RLS can be seen in association with many different conditions, and patients frequently present to neurology, gerontology, rheumatology, hematology and psychiatry in the first instance. However, the bulk of cases are still seen by general practitioners and it is important that they should be familiar with the condition. There is a general lack of robust studies exploring the relationship between RLS and depression, daytime somnolence and pain, as well as the impact of the condition on quality of life, with many physicians considering RLS to be a 'second-line' disorder that patients must 'put up with'.

However, while RLS itself is not life threatening, the implications of years of neglected diagnosis and lack of treatment can manifest as serious depression and even suicidal tendencies in the unfortunate patients. The misfortune of the situation is further compounded by the fact that diagnosis is easy to perform and does not require sophisticated tests and effective treatments are now available that can provide dramatic benefit to many individuals

In this book we present various facets of this fascinating condition, and try to shed light on the causes, epidemiology, differential diagnosis and treatment of RLS. We have tried to be as evidence-based as possible and are fortunate in having several international authorities who have contributed to the chapters.

We hope this book will be useful to specialists, general practitioners and trainees who will no doubt be asked to see patients with RLS more commonly in the future as the awareness of the condition and its treatment grows.

We are grateful to our many colleagues who have contributed to this book and who continue to keep us up to date on the rapid advances in our understanding of the cause, pathogenesis and treatment of RLS.

K. Ray Chaudhuri
Per Odin
C. Warren Olanow

Foreword

I vividly recall reviewing with my group at Johns Hopkins many sleep recordings with excessive leg movements in sleep and routinely diagnosing periodic limb movement disorder of sleep (PLMD), not restless legs syndrome (RLS). That was 1988, less than 20 years ago. We, virtually all of us in sleep medicine, failing to look at wake as closely as sleep and never noticed the marked sensory complaints of RLS. In over a quarter century of running a major sleep center I had not seen one diagnosis of RLS, but lots of PLMD. At about that time I conducted a sobering review of patient satisfaction, finding dismal treatment satisfaction for patients we had labeled PLMD. They were frustrated as were we. Some significant timely events pointed us in a new direction. The serendipitous finding of Akpinar that RLS responded well to dopaminergic treatment and Montplaisir's confirmation of this called our attention to this sensory disorder of waking with its profound motor sign expressed in sleep as periodic leg movements. Almost at the same time our movement disorder colleagues Art Walters and Wayne Hening called attention to the clinical significance of RLS and the effectiveness of opioid treatment. We had been ignoring a medical condition that could now be addressed. Our studies comparing opioid and dopaminergic treatment demonstrated the advantages of the latter. Attending to wake symptoms, as well as the movements in sleep, we could now provide effective treatment.

What a difference the past 20 years has meant for our patients. Patients for years had been told to keep a stiff upper lip; to suffer with their RLS symptoms. The dread of the night-walking, tossing and turning, the agony of trying to sit still in a theatre or plane, the confusion and fatigue with little sleep, all to be tolerated or fear being called crazy. Here was a large unmet medical need. When we offered treatment the patients' response overwhelmed us. I think none of us realized the large number suffering with RLS or appreciated the degree of their suffering that could now be relieved. The patients themselves organized in the United States their Restless Legs Syndrome foundation to increase awareness and promote better treatment. In North America I have been privileged to work with this foundation to help it establish itself. Dr Chaudhuri, the first editor of this book, has taken a similar leading role for the Ekbom support group in the United Kingdom and he knows our experience: patients wrestling treatment for a better life from a somewhat reluctant medical establishment rather than the doctors rushing to their aid. This must change. We must help medical professionals learn about RLS, how to treat and diagnose rather than avoid and minimize RLS.

This book as the first modern medical text on RLS serves the change in medical practice required for better treatment of RLS patients. It provides in one place a readable and comprehensive access to the relevant information about RLS. Health-care professionals will find here the information needed to provide good care for their patients. It should be studied to learn about RLS and it should be used as a basic reference for anyone treating RLS, particularly for doctors providing adult primary care.

I have often been asked why now? If RLS is such a common and significant medical need, why was it ignored for so long? Willis, famous for his discovery of sugar in the urine of diabetics and the circle of arteries at the base of the brain, the circle of Willis, also first described RLS in the medical literature in the 17th century. Then it appeared to be considered an unusual, but not trivial, disorder. Willis living a normal life span for that time died at age 54. While, as noted in this book, RLS may start at any age, it most commonly does not become daily or severely disrupting to life until age 45–60, or about the age Willis died. RLS, when it starts early in life often slowly worsens but it also starts later in life as almost immediately severe. Thus RLS is both a disease of aging and a disease of the aged. This, like many other disorders, becomes a significant medical problem only with the social and medical successes in prolonging life and the associated changing emphasis in medicine toward ensuring good health to promote quality of life as well as longevity. A second major reason for the rediscovery of RLS, has been the development of sleep medicine as a new medical specialty. This called our attention to disorders that disrupt the nighttime. RLS happens to be perhaps the greatest chronic thief of sleep. Untreated, the severe RLS patient gets about 5 hours or less sleep a night, night after night without relief. So the rediscovery of RLS occurs as a natural success of the modern developments of both geriatric and sleep medicine. This good medical book covering this disorder is certainly timely.

Richard P. Allen PhD
Diplomate American Board of Sleep Medicine
Johns Hopkins University
Baltimore, Maryland, USA

1   What is restless legs syndrome?

K. Ray Chaudhuri and C. Meilak

Restless legs syndrome (RLS) is possibly one of the commonest movement disorders known, but remains relatively under-recognized and under-treated within the neurology and movement disorders communities. RLS has been referred to as 'the most common disorder you have ever heard of' by the American Restless Legs Syndrome Foundation. The under-recognition of RLS may be because it is largely perceived as: (a) a disorder of sleep, and (b) a condition with little effective treatment. All of the above assumptions are erroneous and, in the UK, many patients with this condition continue to suffer in spite of effective treatment being available. On the other hand, many are diagnosed inappropriately with RLS when they may have alternative conditions, the so-called RLS 'mimics'. Although RLS principally affects sleep and causes 'terrible nights' and chronic sleeplessness, it also occurs during quiet wakefulness and can affect the hands. It is worth noting that restlessness of legs or arms can be caused by several conditions and these conditions, such as leg cramps, positional discomfort of the legs or pain in the legs, are not the same as RLS, which is a distinct condition in its own right.

Restless legs syndrome is a chronic condition which results in discomfort or pain in the legs and occasionally in the arms and trunk, causing the sufferer much distress and impacting on the ability to sleep. Specific criteria for diagnosis are available and have been widely validated and are extremely simple to administer. The diagnosis of RLS is made clinically and relies on the patient meeting criteria originally set out by the International Restless Legs Syndrome Study Group (IRLSSG). These were further revised in a consensus conference held at the National Institutes of Health in Bethesda, Maryland, USA, May 1–3, 2002[1]. These will be discussed in later chapters.

The prevalence of RLS and periodic limb movements during sleep (PLMS) amongst Caucasians has been estimated at 9–29% and appears to increase with age, although the onset of RLS occurs before the age of 20 in up to 43% of cases, despite the fact that most people present after the age of 50 and may even be wrongly diagnosed as having 'growing pains' or 'hyperactivity' earlier in life. Although the prevalence figures in the UK have not been established, it has been estimated that there may be over 5 million people with RLS. Not all sufferers will have a debilitating form of the disease, but about 20% of sufferers do have a severe form and may be so badly distressed that, as a result of lack of treatment or failure of diagnosis, they may contemplate suicide. This is made even more worrying if we consider that it is not uncommon for people to have suffered for 10 years before a diagnosis is made. It has been suggested that a combination of the patient's reluctance to seek medical advice associated with simply coping with the discomfort or with difficulty in explaining their symptoms, coupled with the lack of adequate treatment until relatively recently, are to blame for the apparent ignorance of RLS. Another contributory factor may be the fact that in itself it is a harmless condition, in the sense that it poses no great threat to life and, unfortunately, this has led to the impact on quality of life being overlooked.

The overall impact of chronic under-treated RLS on sleep function, daytime alertness, mood, cognitive function and quality of life is still largely unknown, even though in the UK alone there may be over 5 million sufferers. Complicating the under-recognition of RLS is the fact that RLS is often paroxysmal.

THE HISTORY OF RESTLESS LEGS SYNDROME

Although recognized in the seventeenth century, the modern history of RLS started with the term 'restless leg syndrome' being coined by Professor Karl-Axel Ekbom in 1945[2,3]. To honor this fact, RLS is also known as 'Ekbom disease'. Ekbom was born in 1907 in Gothenburg in Sweden. He studied medicine at the Karolinska Institute and later became the first professor and head of the department of neurology at Uppsala University Hospital. In his classic 1945 publication[3] entitled *Restless Legs*, Ekbom described the disease and presented eight cases. The addition of the word 'syndrome' to the title of the disorder highlights how the disorder is defined by clinical symptoms rather than by a specific pathological process.

Although Ekbom identified and characterized the syndrome of restless legs, he was probably not the first to describe the disease. The earliest documentation of what was very likely to be RLS occurred some 300 years earlier and is credited to the famous English physician, Thomas Willis[4] (1621–75), who served King Charles II. The son of a small farmer, he studied at the private school of Edward Sylvester in Oxford and worked in the disciplines of anatomy, physiology, medicine, iatrochemistry and

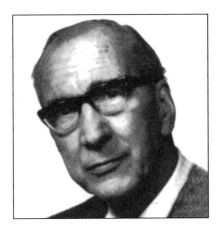

Figure 1.1 Karl-Axel Ekbom (1907–77)

pharmacology. Willis is probably most famous for his publication '*Cerebri Anatome: cui Acessit Nervorum Descriptio et Usus*', published in 1664, which was a fundamental text on the anatomy of the cerebral system.

As Sedleian Professor at Oxford, Willis lectured on physiology; he also identified diabetes mellitus, meningitis and epidemic typhoid fever (1659). This highly accomplished man, amongst numerous other things, also described a case, in 1672, of what might have been RLS using the current diagnostic criteria. Willis wrote in a chapter entitled 'Instructions for curing the Watching evil' in the *London Practice of Physick* (1685):

'*...Wherefore to some, when being in bed they betake themselves to sleep, presently in the arms and legs. Leaping and contractions of the tendons and so great a restlessness and tossing of the members ensure, that the diseased are no more able to sleep, than if they were in the place of the greatest torture...*'

Willis went on to think that the disease originated in the spinal cord and was a product of spinal irritation and used opiates as his therapy of choice. He wrote:

'*Sometimes since I was advised with for a lady of quality, who in the night was hindered from sleep by reason of these spasmodic effects which came upon her only twice a week; she took afterward daily for almost three months, receiving no injury thereby, either on the brain or about any other function, and when while by the use of other remedies; the dyscrasia of the blood and nervous juice being corrected, the animal spirits became more benign and mild. She afterward leaving wholly the opium was able to sleep indifferently well!*'

Willis thought that the cure for RLS was bloodletting, but with modern understanding we know that anemia, iron deficiency and/or low ferritin levels can contribute to RLS.

In the nineteenth century the term 'anxietas tibiarum' was the name given to the condition in Germany and it was believed to be a form of hysteria, whilst in France the term 'impatience musculaire' was adopted.

Descriptions of the disease were also documented by Wittmaak[5] in Germany in 1861 as:

> 'A characteristic feeling is that from older anxietas tibiarum: a strange but descriptive compulsion to move has invaded the legs of the inflicted person. Every moment sees the legs brought into a different position; drawn up, stretched out, abducted, spread apart and crossed over one another. However, these movements are not sudden or violent, rather they are slow, mindful as if it were of eventually finding the one position that will give the most relief. In every strange description of the nervous tension of hysteria one often also finds this train of involuntary agitation displayed in the legs and feet. The same thing also occurs however else where without one being able to find a definite cause...the condition lasts approximately a quarter of an hour.'

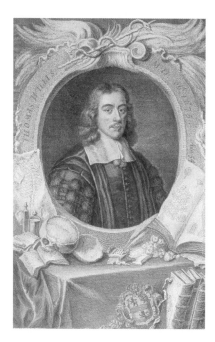

Figure 1.2 Thomas Willis (1621–75)

Beard[6] published an article entitled 'Neurasthenia, or nervous exhaustion' in the *Boston Medical Journal* in 1869. He described the disease as 'one of the myriad results of spinal irritation', suggesting that the spinal cord might be involved from an early stage. In 1923, Oppenheim was the first to describe RLS as a neurological disorder in his *Lehrbuch der Nervenkrankheiten*[7]. His description was also important, as the familial component of the disease was also recognized:

> '*Restlessness in the legs is a special kind of subjective paralgesia. It can become an agonizing torture, lasting for years or decades and can be passed on and occur in other members of the family.*'

In 1940, Mussio-Fournier and Rawak described a 'curious case' of RLS, entitling the disorder a 'familial occurrence of pruritus, urticaria and parasthetic hyperkinesia syndrome of the lower limbs'[8]. However, this particular analysis failed to identify the difference between RLS symptoms and an additional allergic disorder which existed concomitantly in this particular family.

Ekbom himself first described the disease in 1944[2] as:

> '*Asthenia crurum paraesthetica (irritable legs). A new syndrome consisting of weakness, sensation of cold and nocturnal paraesthesia in legs, responding to a certain extent to treatment with priscol and doryl*'[2].

In a later paper[3], published in 1945, he wrote:

> '*A clinical study of a hitherto overlooked disease in the legs, characterized by peculiar paraesthesia, pain and weakness and occurring in two main forms, aestheia crurum paraesthetica and asthenia dolorosa*'.

The differentiation of RLS in these two phenotypically distinct forms is still valid. The emphasis of the description Ekbom gave of this disorder shifted from the previous preoccupation with the movement abnormality alone to the sensory aspect of the disease. Ekbom had made the distinction that the presentation of the disease could vary, although we know that patients will describe a wide variety of sensations other than the clear-cut 'two forms' Ekbom first described.

It is also interesting that Ekbom himself described this disease as 'overlooked', since there is a lack of awareness of this condition. Ekbom was also the first to estimate prevalence of the disorder in a study conducted when he was at the Neurological Department of the Serafimer Hospital, Stockholm[9]. He found that more than 5% of middle-aged people suffered from RLS, and noted a slight preponderance in women. A further estimation of the prevalence of RLS came at the beginning of the 1960s from another Swedish neurologist named Strang[10], at the Karolinska Hospital. However, his methods may have led to an underestimation of the disease.

The link between iron and RLS was formally made in 1953 when Nils Brage Nordlander, a contemporary of Ekbom, put forward the theory that iron insufficiency caused RLS. This differed from Ekbom's emphasis on vascular problems being more important than low levels of iron in the pathogenesis of RLS. Nordlander[11] conducted an open label study on 22 patients and used very large doses of intravenous iron to treat them. Twenty-one of these patients had complete relief from all their symptoms for several months. Of late, most of the pioneering work in relation to iron and RLS has been carried out within the group led by Professor Richard Allen at the Johns Hopkins University, USA[12].

HISTORICAL ASPECTS OF THE ASSOCIATION BETWEEN PERIODIC LIMB MOVEMENT AND RLS

In 1953, Symonds[13] described night-time leg jerking as 'nocturnal myoclonus', which is to some extent a misnomer as the quality of movements may not be typically 'myoclonic' in nature. Lugaresi and colleagues from Italy addressed the issue of what he still called 'nocturnal myoclonus' about 25 years later, commenting on its periodic nature. Lugaresi and colleagues[14] reported that most of their patients with RLS had these periodic movements whilst sleeping, as measured during physiological recordings of sleep. In his study group, 80% of those with RLS had repetitive slow flexion of the limbs, legs, knees and ankles (now defined as periodic limb movements) occurring in stages 1 and 2 of sleep.

It was Coleman[15], a contemporary of Lugaresi, who described the more general association of these limb movements with sleep and the link with sleep disturbance. The term 'periodic limb movements during sleep' (PLMS), has replaced the term nocturnal myoclonus and, although it does indeed occur in those with RLS, it is a separate entity from RLS. Indeed PLMS may occur without the existence of RLS, and Montplaisir[16] relatively recently extended the definition of PLMS to include movements which occur during restful waking and may involve the hands (hence periodic limb movements, not leg movements). It is best, therefore, to use the term PLM rather than PLMS. Whereas RLS remains a clinical diagnosis, PLMS requires polysomnography for its diagnosis.

REFERENCES

1. Walters AS. Toward a better definition of restless legs syndrome. The International Restless Legs Syndrome Study Group. *Mov Disord* 1995;10: 634–42

2. Ekbom KA. Asthenia crurum pasasthetica (irritable legs). *Acta Med Scand* 1944;118:197–209

3. Ekbom KA. Restless Legs Syndrome. *Acta Med Scand* 1945:158 (Suppl);4–122

4. Willis T. *The London Practice of Physick.* London: Basset & Crooke, 1685

5. Wittmaak T. Pathologie und Therapie des Sensibilitäts-Neurosen. *Lehrbuch der Nervenkrankheiten, Teil 1: Pathologie und Therapie der sensiblen Neurosen.* Leipzig: E. Schäfer, 1861

6. Beard GM. Neurasthenia, or nervous exhaustion. *Boston Med J* 1869;80:217–21

7. Oppenheim H. *Lehrbruch der Nervenkranheiten,* 7th edn. Berlin: Karger, 1923: 1774

8. Mussio-Fournier JC, Rawak F. Familiares Auftreten von Prurotus. Urtikaria and parasthetischer Hyerkinese der unteren Extremitaten. *Confin Neurol* 1940;3: 110–15

9. Ekbom KA. Restless legs syndrome. *Neurology* 1960;10:868–73

10. Strang RR. The symptoms of restless legs. *Med J Aust* 1967;1:1211–13

11. Nordlander NB. Therapy in restless legs. *Acta Med Scand* 1953;143:453–7

12. Allen RP, Barker PB, Wehrl F, *et al.* MRI measurement of brain iron in patients with restless legs syndrome. *Neurology* 2001;56:263–5

13. Symonds CP. Nocturnal myoclonus. *J Neurochem* 1953;16:166–71

14. Lugaresi E, Coccagna G, Tassinari CA, Ambrosetto C. Polygraphic data on motor phenomena in the restless legs syndrome [In Italian]. *Riv Neurol* 1965;35(6):550–61

15. Coleman R. Periodic movements in sleep (nocturnal myoconus) and restless legs syndrome. In Guilleminault C, ed. *Sleeping and Waking Disorders: Indications and Techniques.* Menlo Park, CA: Addison-Wesley, 1982:265–95

16. Montplaisir J, Boucher S, Poirier G, *et al.* Clinical, polysomnographic, and genetic characteristics of restless legs syndrome: a study of 133 patients diagnosed with new standard criteria. *Mov Disord* 1997;12:61–5

2

Diagnostic criteria

P. Odin

The diagnosis of RLS is mainly based on the patient's clinical history[1,2]. In patients with typical symptoms, the diagnosis is easy. However, it can be difficult in patients with either atypical symptomatology or co-morbidity, for example with other sleep or movement disorders. The diagnosis of RLS is based on criteria proposed by a consensus conference held at the National Institutes of Health, May 1–3, 2002, in Bethesda, Maryland, USA[2]. These criteria are essentially based on criteria published by the International Restless Legs Syndrome Study Group, IRLSSG[1], and represent an update of these as a result of the improved understanding of the disease. Allen and colleagues also developed new criteria for the diagnosis of RLS in the cognitively impaired elderly (Tables 2.3 and 2.4) and in children (Tables 2.5–2.8). The consensus conference also suggested diagnostic criteria for RLS augmentation (Table 2.9).

THE ESSENTIAL CRITERIA FOR RLS

1. *An urge to move the legs, usually accompanied or caused by uncomfortable or unpleasant sensations in the legs. (Sometimes the urge to move is present without the uncomfortable sensations and sometimes the arms or other body parts are involved in addition to the legs.)*

The most typical clinical presentation is when the patients talk about their inability to remain at rest and about a pronounced discomfort if they are forced to stay at rest. This is an urgent internal sense that the body part, usually one or more of the limbs, must be moved. When pronounced, this can be a feeling that the whole body needs to be moved, but it always contains a component of having to move a specific body part, most often the legs. This is usually (but not always) associated with unpleasant sensations (a deep sense of movement inside the limb) and the diagnostic criteria demand that if the sensations occur they should be linked to the urge to move. The discomfort is often described in terms such as: 'creeping, crawling, itching, burning, searing, tugging, pulling, drawing, aching, heat/coldness, electric current-like, restlessness or pain' and seems to be located deep

Table 2.1   Diagnostic criteria for diagnosis of idiopathic restless legs syndrome (RLS) according to a 2002 NIH-supported workshop on RLS diagnosis

Essential diagnostic criteria

1.   An urge to move the legs, usually accompanied or caused by uncomfortable or unpleasant sensations in the legs. (Sometimes the urge to move is present without the uncomfortable sensations and sometimes the arms or other body parts are involved in addition to the legs.)

2.   The urge to move or unpleasant sensations begin or worsen during periods of rest or inactivity such as lying or sitting

3.   The urge to move or unpleasant sensations are partially or totally relieved by movement, such as walking or stretching, at least as long as the activity continues

4.   The urge to move or unpleasant sensations are worse in the evening or night than during the day or only occur in the evening or night. (When symptoms are very severe, the worsening at night may not be noticeable but must have been previously present.)

Supportive of the diagnosis

1.   Family history

2.   Response to dopaminergic therapy

3.   Periodic limb movements (during wakefulness or sleep)

Associated features

1.   Natural clinical course

2.   Sleep disturbance

3.   Medical evaluation/physical examination

in the muscle or bone, seldom in a joint (Table 2.2). The location of the sensory symptoms in the leg can vary, and occasionally extend to involve the whole lower limb or even the upper limb. Arm symptomatology has been reported in up to half of patients with idiopathic RLS. The involvement of arms without involvement of legs is, however, an exception[3–5]. The symptoms can occur unilaterally or bilaterally.

Table 2.2   Descriptions of RLS sensations in the legs

Aching	Indescribable
Burning	Itching
Coldness	Like Coca-Cola
Crazy legs	Like water flowing
Crawling	Painful
Creeping	Pulling
Drawing	Restless
Electric current	Searing
Elvis legs	Tearing
Gotta-moves	Throbbing
Growing pains	Toothache-like
Heat	Tugging
Heeby-jeebies	

Table 2.3   Essential criteria for the diagnosis of probable RLS in the cognitively impaired elderly (all five are necessary for diagnosis)

1. Signs of leg discomfort such as rubbing or kneading the legs and groaning while holding the lower extremities

2. Excessive motor activity in the lower extremities such as pacing, fidgeting, repetitive kicking, tossing and turning in bed, slapping the legs on the mattress, cycling movements of the lower limbs, repetitive foot tapping, rubbing the feet together and the inability to remain seated

3. Signs of leg discomfort are exclusively present or worsen during periods of rest or inactivity

4. Signs of leg discomfort are diminished with activity

5. Criteria 1 and 2 occur only in the evening or at night or are worse at those times than during the day

2. *The urge to move or unpleasant sensations begin or worsen during periods of rest or inactivity such as lying or sitting.*

The symptoms begin with a delay of some minutes up to 1 hour when the patient is lying or sitting[4]. Rest induces these symptoms independent of prior activity and body position. The more restful the situation is and the

Table 2.4 Supportive or suggestive criteria for the diagnosis of probable RLS in cognitive-impaired elderly

1. Dopaminergic responsiveness

2. Patient's past history – as reported by a family member, caregiver, or friend – is suggestive of RLS

3. A first-degree, biologic relative (sibling, child, or parent) has RLS

4. Observed periodic limb movements while awake or during sleep

5. Periodic limb movements of sleep recorded by polysomnography or actigraphy

6. Significant sleep-onset problems

7. Better quality sleep in the day than at night

8. The use of restraints at night (for institutionalized patients)

9. Low serum ferritin level

10. End-stage renal disease

11. Diabetes

12. Clinical, electromyographic or nerve-conduction evidence of peripheral neuropathy or radiculopathy

longer it continues, the more likely it is that the symptoms appear. Typical situations where the symptoms are present include (apart from lying in bed or sitting in a chair) the passive rest of longer journeys by car, train or plane, as well as visits to meetings, theater and cinema. In advanced cases such activities are almost impossible to perform. The symptoms occur when resting or lying down, not typically only when sitting. The symptoms often become more intense the longer the period of rest continues. Rest is here a matter both of decreased movements and decreased mental alertness.

3. *The urge to move or unpleasant sensations are partially or totally relieved by movement, such as walking or stretching, at least as long as the activity continues.*

The relief normally comes immediately with movement. This immediacy of the relief differs from many other disorders, particularly those involving pain. The body part which is moved must not be the one affected by RLS.

Table 2.5   Criteria for the diagnosis of definite RLS in children

1.	The child meets all four essential criteria for RLS and
2.	The child relates a description in his or her own words that is consistent with leg discomfort (the child may use terms such as 'owies', 'tickle', 'spiders', 'boo-boos', 'want to run' or 'a lot of energy in my legs' to describe symptoms)

or

1.	The child meets all four essential adult criteria and
2.	Two out of the three following supportive criteria are present:
a.	Sleep disturbance for age
b.	A biological parent or sibling has definite RLS
c.	The child has a polysomnographically documented periodic limb movement index of 5 or more per hour of sleep

Table 2.6   Criteria for the diagnosis of probable RLS in children

1.	The child meets all essential adult criteria for RLS, except criterion 4 (the urge to move or sensations are worse in the evening or at night than during the day), and
2.	The child has a biological parent or sibling with definite RLS

or

1.	The child is observed to have behavior manifestations of lower extremity discomfort when sitting or lying, accompanied by motor movement of the affected limb, the discomfort has characteristics of adult criteria 2, 3 and 4 (i.e. is worse during rest and inactivity, relieved by movement, and worse during the evening and at night) and
2.	The child has a biological parent or sibling with definite RLS

Table 2.7   Criteria for the diagnosis of possible RLS in children

1.	The child has periodic limb movement disorder and
2.	The child has a biological parent or sibling with definite RLS, but the child does not meet definite or probable childhood RLS definitions

Table 2.8 Criteria for the diagnosis of PLMD in children (age 0 to 18 years)

1. Polysomnography shows a periodic limb movement index of 5 or more per hour of sleep. The leg movements are 0.5–5 s in duration, occur at intervals of 5–90 s, occur in groups of four or more, and have an amplitude of one-quarter or more of toe dorsiflexion during calibration, and

2. Clinical sleep disturbance for age must be evident as manifest by sleep onset problems, sleep maintenance problems or excessive sleepiness, and

3. The leg movements cannot be accounted for by sleep disordered breathing (i.e. the movements are independent of any abnormal respiratory events) or medication effect (e.g. antidepressant medication)

Table 2.9 Key features of augmentation in RLS

Augmentation is the shifting of symptoms to a period of time 2 h or earlier than the typical time of daily onset of symptoms before pharamcologic intervention

1. An increased overall intensity of the urge to move or of sensation is temporally related to an increase in the daily medication dosage

2. A decreased overall intensity of the urge to move or of sensation is temporally related to a decrease in the daily medication dosage

3. The latency to RLS symptoms at rest is shorter than the latency with initial therapeutic response or before treatment was instituted.

4. The urge to move or sensation is extended to previously unaffected limbs or body parts

5. The duration of treatment effect is shorter than the duration with initial therapeutic response

6. Periodic limb movements while awake either occur for the first time or are worse than with initial therapeutic response or before treatment was instituted

Typically the patient paces the floor, rubs the legs and, stretches and flexes the extremities. The patient feels compelled to move, but the choice of type of movement is voluntary. In mild cases the patient might not have to get up to walk; it might be sufficient to move around in the bed or chair. The relief from movement continues at least as long as the limb is being moved. The relief is not always complete. Symptoms may recur almost immediately when movement stops. Therefore some patients may falsely report that they have no relief from movement. In advanced disease the patient might no longer have much relief from movement, but she/he should then be able to recapitulate that there was, earlier in the disease development, improvement with movements. Instead of movement some patients produce a counter-stimulus, for example heat or cold[6].

4. *The urge to move or unpleasant sensations are worse in the evening or night than during the day or only occur in the evening or night. (When symptoms are very severe, the worsening at night may not be noticeable but must have been previously present.)*

In typical cases, the untreated patient reaches maximal symptomatology between 12 p.m. and 4 a.m. and a maximal relief between 6 and 12 a.m.[7,8]. The night-time worsening occurs whether the patient is sleeping or not. Most patients have a period during the day when the symptoms are much less pronounced. At this time the patients should be able to rest with no or very mild RLS symptoms. In very severe cases, however, the patient experiences the symptoms almost constantly without any circadian rhythm. Mostly such patients can, however, tell about having a circadian pattern earlier in the disease development. A few patients with a rapid onset of a severe RLS might have difficulties identifying any periods of improvement or a circadian rhythm. Patients who have symptoms only during prolonged periods of rest, such as when traveling, might not experience a circadian rhythm. The circadian rhythm can be influenced by medication, but also by shift work, sleep disorders and irregular sleep patterns.

DIAGNOSTIC PROCEDURE

The new criteria include four essential criteria and three supportive clinical features (Table 2.1), the latter describing phenomena occurring frequently although not being strictly necessary for diagnosis. Following a clinical interview, other causes for the symptomatology need to be excluded through clinical examination. If necessary, laboratory tests and neurophysiological investigations are performed. The diagnosis is further supported if there is an improvement of symptoms after dopaminergic medication. A sleep study might be of further help if further diagnostic difficulties are still present. However, in clinical neurological practice sleep studies are not essential for diagnosis of RLS.

Common clinical confounders of RLS, the so called RLS mimics, are nocturnal leg cramps, positional discomfort of legs and drug-induced akathisia.

SUPPORTIVE CLINICAL FEATURES

Apart from the essential diagnostic criteria, there are *supportive clinical features*, including:

1. A family history of RLS

More than 50% of the patients with idiopathic RLS report on family members having the disease. A person with RLS is thereby 3–6 times more likely to have a family history of RLS compared to a person without the disease. There is increasing evidence for an autosomal dominant mode of inheritance[3].

2. A response to dopaminergic therapy

More than 90% of the RLS patients report on initial relief from RLS symptoms with L-dopa and/or dopamine agonists. The doses needed for effect are comparatively low (relative to the doses needed in Parkinson's disease). These effects have been well documented in a large number of controlled and non-controlled clinical studies (see treatment section).

3. Periodic limb movements (PLM) (in wakefulness or sleep)

PLMS (PLM in sleep) occur in over 80% of the patients[9], but are not obligatory for diagnosis. PLMS can vary in their pattern, but are often seen as repetitive flexing of lower limb joints (hip, knee or ankle and occasionally the upper limb) and dorsiflexion or fanning of toes. To be scored, these movements should occur in a series of four consecutive movements lasting for periods of 0.5–5 seconds, have an amplitude of one-quarter or more of the toe dorsiflexion during calibration, and are separated by intervals of 4–90 seconds. An index (number of PLMS per hour of sleep) >5 for the entire night is pathological (American Sleep Disorders Association 1993). PLMS are, however, not specific for RLS, but occur in a number of diseases, medical conditions and also normally, especially in elderly people. PLMS (as also PLM during waking time, PLMW) are, however, more frequent in

RLS. An elevated PLMS index is therefore supportive of RLS diagnosis and a patient without PLMS is unlikely to have RLS.

ASSOCIATED FEATURES OF RLS

Apart from the diagnostic criteria, the following characteristics are typical:

1. Natural clinical course

RLS can occur at any age. Early onset suggests hereditary RLS and late onset suggests secondary RLS. Typically the symptomatology initially is fluctuating, later becoming a continuous or chronic-progressive course[10]. Remissions might occur, and especially in mild cases the symptoms can also permanently disappear. Secondary RLS can disappear when the cause of the symptoms disappears (renal transplantation, end of pregnancy). Early-onset RLS often develops slowly over many years, and late adult-onset RLS often has a more rapid course[11,12].

2. Sleep disturbance

More than 90% of patients report difficulties initiating or maintaining sleep. Sleep problems are often the primary reason why the patient seeks medical help. In sleep laboratory investigations it was possible to verify increased sleep latency and PLMs-associated arousals/awakenings, along with a decrease in total sleep time, sleep efficiency and slow-wave sleep. The sleep efficiency is often reduced below 50% of normal. Patients with moderate–severe RLS often have < 5 hours of sleep per night[13].

3. Medical evaluation/physical examination

The neurological examination is typically normal in both primary and secondary forms of RLS. Patients with late-onset disease might, however, show signs for radiculopathy or neuropathy. The main aim of the examination is to identify possible primary causes for secondary RLS (pregnancy, renal disease, iron deficiency).

DIAGNOSTIC CRITERIA FOR RLS IN COGNITIVELY IMPAIRED ELDERLY AND CHILDREN

The NIH workshop members[2] have recently suggested new criteria for the diagnosis of RLS in patients where the use of traditional criteria is less suitable, namely cognitively impaired elderly and children. These criteria are summarized in Tables 2.1–2.6.

For cognitively-impaired elderly, the difficulty getting adequate verbal information from the patient has motivated criteria that are more based on behavioral indicators (excessive motor activity, use of counterstimulus), supportive features and history from family members and caregivers (Tables 2.3 and 2.4).

Also, children might describe and exhibit RLS symptoms differently compared to grown-ups[3]. The occurrence of RLS in children is well documented and RLS in this case often seems related to sleep disturbance and neurobehavioral problems. This is an area where further studies are of high interest and this has prompted the publication of separate consensus criteria for diagnosis in children (Tables 2.5–2.8). The definite RLS criteria are aimed at children between the ages of 2 and 12. To avoid over-diagnosing, these criteria have been formulated more strictly than the adult criteria, demanding both urge to move and leg discomfort for diagnosis. From 13 years of age the adult criteria are recommended.

The workshop has also developed criteria for PLMD in children (Table 2.8; for ages 0–18 years). The relation between PLMD and RLS in children is still not clear and the two should be regarded as separate but related phenomena. The prevalence and clinical significance of PLMD in children are still unknown.

DIAGNOSTIC CRITERIA FOR AUGMENTATION IN RLS

Augmentation has been found to be a common problem for dopaminergic treatments of RLS. Augmentation has been defined as a shifting of RLS symptoms to a period of time 2 hours or earlier than was the typical period of daily onset of symptoms before pharmacologic intervention. If this is not the case, augmentation may also be diagnosed if therapy results in two or more of the key features that are listed in Table 2.5. The augmentation symptoms should be present for at least 1 week, for a minimum of 5 days per week, to meet diagnostic criteria. In a study by Allen and Earley[13], 82% of patients using L-dopa developed augmentation. The risk for augmentation seems to be lower when using dopamine agonists (see therapy section).

Rebound, another problem in the dopaminergic treatment, is characterized by the development of RLS symptoms in the early morning, rather than by earlier onset of symptoms in the evening, and is thought to represent an end-of-dose effect[14]. Rebound seems to occur more seldom (20%) and seems to be less of a clinical problem compared to augmentation.

SUMMARY OF PRACTICAL QUESTIONS TO ASK THE RLS SUFFERER

Taking a good clinical history so as to exclude the RLS mimics is essential, and the following questions are provided as a guide for the inexperienced investigator to aid diagnosis of RLS in patients. Ask if:

- The pattern of leg disturbance is diurnal? Are their symptoms specifically worse at night?

- Do their limb symptoms become more troublesome during quiet restfulness, for example sitting down to watch a film or television?

- Do they have the urge to move around and does doing so ease their discomfort?

- If they are distracted (physically or mentally) do the symptoms improve?

- Are any of the sensations worse if they are in contact with the bedclothes?

- Have they suffered from disrupted sleep and/or do they feel sleepy during the day?

REFERENCES

1. Walters AS. International Restless Legs Syndrome Study Group. Towards a better definition of restless legs syndrome. *Mov Disord* 1995;10:634–42

2. Allen RP, Picchietti D, Wayne AH, *et al*. The participants in the Restless Legs Syndrome Diagnosis and Epidemiology workshop at the National Institutes of Health in collaboration with members of the International Restless Legs Syndrome Study Group. Restless legs syndrome: diagnostic criteria, special considerations, and epidemiology. *Sleep Med* 2003;4:101–19

3. Winkelmann J, Muller-Myhsok B, Wittchen HU, *et al*. Complex segregation analysis of restless legs syndrome provides evidence for an autosomal dominant mode of inheritance in early age at onset families. *Ann Neurol* 2002;52:297–302

4. Michaud M, Lavigne G, Desautels A, *et al*. Effects of immobility on sensory and motor symptoms of restless legs syndrome. *Mov Disord* 2002;17:112–25

5. Fukunishi I, Kitaoka T, Shirai T, Kino K. Facial paresthesias resembling restless legs syndrome in a patient on hemodialysis. *Nephron* 1998;79:485

6. Winkelmann J, Wetter TC, Collado-Seidel V, *et al*. Clinical characteristics and frequency of the hereditary restless legs syndrome in a population of 300 patients. *Sleep* 2000;23:597–602

7. Hening WA, Walters AS, Wagner M, *et al*. Circadian rhythm of motor restlessness and sensory symptoms in the idiopathic restless legs syndrome. *Sleep* 1999;22:901–12

8. Trenkwalder C, Hening WA, Walters AS, *et al*. Circadian rhythm of periodic limb movements and sensory symptoms of restless legs syndrome. *Mov Disord* 1999;14:102–10

9. Montplaisir J, Boucher S, Poirier G, *et al*. Clinical, polysomnographic, and genetic characteristics of restless legs syndrome: A study of 133 patients diagnosed with the new standard criteria. *Mov Disord* 1997;12:61–5

10. Walters AS, Hickey K, Maltzmann J, *et al*. A questionnaire study of 138 patients with restless legs syndrome: The 'Night-Walkers' survey. *Neurology* 1996;46:92–5

11. Allen RP, Earley CJ. Defining the phenotype of the restless legs syndrome (RLS) using age-of-symptom-onset. *Sleep Med* 2000;1:11–19

12. Housman D, Gephardt S, Earley C, Allen R. Critical age for development of daily restless leg syndrome symptoms. *Sleep* 2001;24:A355

13. Allen RP, Earley CJ. Restless legs syndrome: a review of clinical and pathophysiologic features. *J Clin Neurophysiol* 2001;18:128–47

14. Guilleminault C, Cetel M, Philip P. Dopaminergic treatment of restless legs and rebound phenomenon. *Neurology* 1993;43:445

15. The Atlas Task Force. Recording and scoring leg movements. *Sleep* 1993;16:748–59

3

Epidemiology

M. Jöbges, P. Odin and K. Ray Chaudhuri

Ekbom himself estimated a 5% prevalence of RLS in the general population[1], whereas later studies have reported prevalences varying between 1.2% and 29% . Thus data on the epidemiology of RLS are variable and this may be due to several possible reasons. In 1995, the International Restless Legs Syndrome Study Group (IRLSSG) published a consensus report for the diagnosis of RLS[2] (see Chapter 2). There are very few large studies (including more than 100 participants) using these criteria. This may be because the investigators used only a few questions[3], or because the surveys were performed before the publication of the 1995 criteria for RLS.

Not only different diagnostic criteria, but also different strategies of data collection may influence the results. Using questionnaires is often the simplest way to reach high numbers of participants, but different participants interpret the questions in different ways. Telephone interviews are more precise, but also more time-consuming and expensive; for this reason only smaller populations can be reached. Face-to-face interviews and examinations by RLS-trained physicians are the most time-consuming and expensive, but are the most sensitive and specific way to acquire the data.

Furthermore, the selection of the study population has to be taken into account. Are the studies based on clinical patient populations or on the general population? It is quite obvious that these aspects influence the results of epidemiological studies. To enable the readers to build up their own opinions, the above aspects will, together with the results, be discussed in detail in the following sections.

PREVALENCE – STUDIES ON GENERAL POPULATIONS

Only a few studies are based on the general population. We have selected three large investigations carried out in Canada, the USA and Europe. A survey conducted through personal interviews was performed in Canada to estimate the prevalence of subjective symptoms related to RLS and to sleep bruxism. Of the 2019 respondents, all over 18 years of age, 15% reported leg restlessness at bedtime; 10% reported unpleasant leg muscle sensations associated with awakenings during sleep and with an irresistible need to move or walk. These questions cover two of the four criteria of the IRLSSG definition of RLS, so probably the prevalence applying the full definition is lower[4].

A question reflecting clinical features of RLS was added to the 1996 Kentucky Behavioral Risk Factor Surveillance. Data were collected by telephone interview from 1803 men and women, 18 years of age and older. The prevalence of RLS for Kentucky adults was 10.0%[3]. The concrete question was: 'Do you have unpleasant feelings in your legs – for example creepy-crawling or tingly feelings – when you lie down at night, that make you feel restless and keep you from getting a good night's sleep?' Restless legs syndrome was considered to be present if restless legs symptoms were reported to occur more than five times per month. The original question is cited to illustrate the limitations of this study. It covers only two of the four criteria of the IRLSSG definition and so it is likely that the estimated prevalence of RLS for Kentucky adults is probably under 10.0%.

Ohayon and Rort[5] reported on cross-sectional studies performed in the UK, Germany, Italy, Portugal and Spain. Overall, 18980 subjects aged 15–100 years, representative of the general populations of these five European countries, underwent telephone interviews with the Sleep-EVAL system. The diagnosis of RLS was based on the minimal criteria provided by the International Classification of Sleep Disorders (ICSD). The prevalence of RLS within this definition was 5.5%. The ICSD definition employs three criteria: (1) a complaint of unpleasant sensation in the legs at night or difficulties in initiating sleep; (2) disagreeable sensations of 'creeping' inside the calves often associated with general aches and pains in the legs; (3) the discomfort is relieved by movements of the limbs. A minor limitation of this definition may be that it is focussed on the sleep-disturbing character of RLS. A diagnostic advantage is the exclusion of sleep disorders that cause similar symptoms in the last step of the interview. In conclusion, the estimated prevalence of 5.5% for European adults seems to be reliable[5] (Table 3.1). Interestingly, this figure is very similar to Ekbom's estimation of a prevalence of 5% for the general population in 1960[1].

CONTRIBUTING FACTORS

Age

The three above-mentioned studies also investigated the age-dependency of RLS. In the Canadian study the prevalence of RLS increased linearly with age. The prevalence increased from 9% and 5% (positive answers to

Table 3.1 Prevalence of RLS

First author	Year published	Country performed	Number of participants	Prevalence found (%)
Ekbom	1945	Sweden	529	5.2
Strang	1967	Sweden	320	2.5
Lavigne	1994	Canada	2019	10–15
Phillips	2000	USA	1803	10
Schmitt	2000	Switzerland	1473	4
Rothdach	2000	Germany	369	9.8
Tan	2001	Singapore	1157	0.1–0.6
Ulfberg	2001	Sweden	200 (women)	11.4
Ulfberg	2001	Sweden	4000 (men)	5.8
Ohayon	2002	Europe	18 980	5.5

questions 1 and 2, respectively) in the 18–29-year-old age group to 23% and 18%, respectively, in the > 60-year-old group. In Kentucky, 3% of participants aged 18–29 years, 10% of those aged 30–70 years and 19% of those aged 80 years and older experienced RLS. Ohayon calculated odds ratios (OR) with age as variable. The OR increased from 0.81 in the 20–29-year-old age group to 1.72 in the > 80-year-old age group.

Ulfberg and co-workers sent a questionnaire to 4000 men living in central Sweden including questions about sleep habits, symptoms of sleepiness and somatic and neuropsychiatric complaints. Four symptom questions, accepted as minimal diagnostic criteria for RLS, were also included. A total of 5.8% of the men suffered from RLS. The prevalence of RLS increased with age, being 1.2% between 18 and 24, 4.0% between 25 and 34, 6.2% between 35 and 44, 8.0% between 45 and 54 and 10.5% between 55 and 64 years of age[6]. In 2000, Rothdach and co-workers published a paper dealing with a population-based survey of the elderly (German population 65–83 years of age) using standard diagnostic criteria of the IRLSSG. Two RLS-trained physicians assessed the prevalence of RLS using standardized questions in face-to-face interviews. They also performed a standardized neurological examination for each participant. The study population included

369 participants; they identified 9.8% as being RLS-positive[7]. In conclusion, a correlation of prevalence between RLS and age seems likely.

A few studies focus on the age of onset of RLS. In 1997 Montplaisir[8] studied 133 RLS patients diagnosed with the IRLSSG criteria by questionnaire and with all-night polysomnographic recordings. Results showed that RLS started at a mean age of 27.2 years and before the age of 20 in 38.3% of patients. Symptoms often appeared in one leg only and also involved upper limbs in about half of all cases.

Walters and co-workers[9] conducted a survey of age of onset of 107 adult patients with RLS. Of the sample, 19.6% had an age of onset between 0 and 10 years and 23.4% had an age of onset between 11 and 20 years. However, those with age of onset < 20 years did not seek medical attention until an average of 32 years of age, and a correct diagnosis was not made until an average of 50 years. Two years later a study concerning the same topic was published by Walters and co-workers. In 105 patients who were part of a nationwide support group, a telephone survey of their symptomatology was undertaken. The answers were compared with those of 33 of the authors' own RLS patients who had undergone a neurological examination. The diagnostic criteria of the IRLSSG were used. Of the patients, 12–20% experienced the onset of RLS below the age of 10; 25% experienced the onset between 11 and 20 years. There was a relatively even distribution of onset of symptoms across the other decades up to the age of 60 years (6–15%). Incorrect diagnosis or failure to make a diagnosis was common and patients had to wait for an average 2 years after first seeking medical attention before a correct diagnosis was made. A remission of symptoms of 1 month or more occurred in at least 15% of the individuals in all patient groups[10].

In summary, there is a correlation between age and prevalence of RLS, and the age of onset seems to occur during childhood and adolescence in about a quarter of the patients.

Sex

Most epidemiological studies also contain data on the distribution of RLS according to sex. In the population-based Kentucky study prevalence did not vary significantly with sex[11]. In Lavignes' Canadian survey[4] the two RLS-indicating questions were answered positively by, respectively, 13% to 9% of the male and, respectively, 17% to 12% of the female participants. Ohayon states that the prevalence was higher in women than in men (in the corresponding table prevalence in women is 3.6% and in men 7.1%; this contradiction makes a consideration of the data difficult)[5]. The MEMO study found the prevalence of RLS higher in women compared with men (female 13.87%, male 6.12%)[7]. Walters described a prevalence distribution of 42 male and 96 female RLS patients[10].

A study from Ulfberg and co-workers includes women only[12]. A total of 200 women, aged 18–64 years, living in a county in mid-Sweden, were sent a questionnaire that included questions about sleep habits, symptoms of sleepiness and neuropsychiatric complaints. IRLSSG criteria were used; 11.4% of the women suffered from RLS[12]. In a parallel study of 4000 men aged 18–64 years the same authors found that 5.8% of the men suffered from RLS[6]. In summary there seems to be some evidence for a female preponderance in the prevalence of RLS.

FAMILY HISTORY

Ekbom stated in 1944: 'However, crawling sensations in the legs occur so often in relatives of persons with asthenia crurum paraesthetica that there is decided reason to believe in the existence of definite hereditary factors'.

Fifty-six years later Winkelmann and co-workers[14] conducted a study confirming this observation. To assess the frequency and characteristics of hereditary RLS in comparison with those of non-hereditary RLS, they analyzed the clinical data of 330 RLS patients. All 300 patients were diagnosed as having RLS according to the IRLSSG criteria. Family history was rated as definitely positive when at least one first-degree relative was examined and classified as RLS according to the criteria, by one of the authors. If it proved impossible to contact family members to verify reports of a family history, the patients were classified as having a 'possible positive family history'. In all, 232 of 300 patients had idiopathic RLS (iRLS) and 68 had secondary RLS due to uremia (uRLS). Further, 42.3% of the patients with iRLS and 11.7% of those with uRLS were classified as having 'definite positive' hereditary RLS, with a further 12.6% of iRLS and 5.8% of uRLS patients having 'possible positive' hereditary RLS. Patients with definite hereditary RLS were significantly younger at the age of onset than those with a negative family history (35.45 vs. 47.17 years, $p < 0.05$). The clinical characteristics of the disease were similar in both groups, except that women with hereditary RLS experienced a worsening of symptoms during pregnancy (19.1% vs. 2.6%, $p < 0.05$).

Godbout and co-workers[15] delivered another piece of evidence to support Ekbom's statement. Among 22 cases of primary RLS investigated at their center, nine (41%) had a positive family history of RLS and six were included in the reported study. Each family was studied for at least three generations. Data were collected for 209 members of these families and RLS was present in 93 (44.5%). In one family, the propositus had an identical twin sister also affected with RLS. These results suggest that there is a strong genetic contribution to the transmission of RLS. The rate of familial cases of RLS could reach 40–50%.

Ondo and Jankovic[16] studied 54 patients (29 women) who satisfied the IRLSSG diagnostic criteria for RLS. The mean age of the patients was 62.69 years, and the mean age of onset was 34 years. They found that 92% of patients with idiopathic RLS (defined by Ondo as definite RLS without neuropathy) had a family history, whereas only 13% of those with neuropathic RLS (defined as definite RLS associated with peripheral neuropathy) had a positive family history. The sporadic/neuropathic patients were older at symptom onset and tended to have a more rapid progression than the familial/idiopathic patients. There were no other significant differences between the subgroups.

GEOGRAPHICAL ASPECTS

As mentioned before, three general population-based epidemiological studies on prevalence of RLS found similar data, indicating a prevalence between 5% and 10% in the European and North American populations. In the Asian population, RLS seems to be relatively uncommon. Tan and co-workers[17] investigated in face-to-face interviews 157 consecutive individuals aged 55 years and older, selected from the general population of Singapore, and 1000 consecutive individuals aged 21 years and older, from a primary healthcare center. All participants underwent a neurological examination. Based on IRLSSG criteria, the prevalence of restless leg syndrome was 0.6 and 0.1%, respectively. There were limitations to this study: patients with diabetes, hypertension and ischemic heart disease were not included. Therefore the estimated prevalence might be too low, but it is very unlikely that it will reach 5–10%. Recently, Krishnan and colleagues[18] reported a 0.8% rate of RLS among an Indian population. In conclusion, the prevalence of RLS is low in Singapore, and possibly India, supporting a frequently held observation that RLS is relatively uncommon in Asians.

UREMIA/END-STAGE RENAL DISEASE

Already in 1966 Callaghan[19] reported on five patients with RLS out of 20 patients with renal damage, this first anecdotal observation being supported by a large number of later studies. One of the most ambitious was published in 1991 by Rogers and co-workers[20]. They tried to uncover the relevance of anemia, polyneuropathy and treatment with epoetin alfa in connection with end-stage renal disease. Fifty-five patients (mean duration of dialysis 37 months) receiving either hemodialysis ($n = 34$) or continuous ambulatory peritoneal dialysis ($n = 21$) were assessed: 22 patients had RLS (40%, diagnostic criteria not mentioned). RLS was related to duration of dialysis (long vs. short time, $p < 0.01$). Patients with RLS had a lower hemoglobin than those who did not (82 vs. 95 g/l, $p = 0.03$). There was no relation between the presence of RLS and clinical evidence of peripheral neuropathy, or its severity, as assessed clinically by grading of vibration sense and tendon jerks in the legs and feet.

In another group of 27 hemodialysis patients (duration of dialysis 41 months), 11 of whom were among the 55 in the first study, the authors investigated the effect of epoetin alfa (erythropoietin). Before and after 6 and 12 months of epoetin alfa the patients were asked to grade the severity of restless legs from one (not present) to seven (very severe). Seventeen patients had RLS before treatment with epoetin alfa (score 4.1), the symptoms being less severe after 6 months (score 2.3) and 12 months (score 1.9) of treatment. Hemoglobin concentration was 66 g/l before treatment and rose to 99 g/l at 6 months and 96 at 12 months. None of the patients without RLS before epoetin alfa had RLS during the 12 month of treatment. There was no correlation between the presence of the symptoms and initial ferritin concentrations or the subsequent need for iron supplementation.

In these two studies the only association found was between RLS and anemia, and the RLS symptoms improved by correcting the anemia with epoetin alfa. Although this strong association does not prove a causal relation, it suggests that anemia, or some closely related factor, is implicated in the pathogenesis of RLS in uremic patients receiving chronic dialysis. Winkelmann and co-workers[21] found in a survey in 1996 a RLS prevalence of 20% in end-stage renal disease patients. This study used a questionnaire taking three of the four IRLSSG diagnostic criteria into consideration (204 patients were questioned)[21]. RLS, when present, normally persists but is reported to resolve after successful kidney transplantation[22].

In summary, end-stage renal disease involves an increased risk for secondary RLS. The role of renal anemia is still somewhat unclear, but treatment with epoetin alfa and kidney transplantation can have positive effects regarding the RLS symptoms.

ANEMIA/IRON DEFICIENCY

In 1953 Nordlander published a paper on 'Therapy in restless legs', mentioning the positive effect of iron substitution on RLS[23]. This was stressed by Ekbom 7 years later[1]. In 1994 O'Keefe[24] threw more light on the relationship between iron status and RLS. A study was carried out of 18 elderly patients with RLS and 18 matched control subjects. Serum ferritin levels were reduced in the RLS patients compared with control subjects; serum iron, vitamin B_{12} and folate levels and hemoglobin levels did not differ between two groups. Fifteen patients with RLS were treated with ferrous sulfate for 2 months. RLS severity improved in ten of these. Although the authors dealt with small numbers of patients, the following conclusion is possibly justified: iron deficiency, with or without anemia, is an important contributor to the development of RLS in elderly patients, and iron supplements can produce significant reduction in symptoms.

PREGNANCY

Not only in the elderly, but also in pregnancy RLS is a very common condition. Already Ekbom recognized this: "I found the incidence of RLS in pregnant women to be 11%"[1]. Keeping this in mind, Ekbom estimated the prevalence of RLS in the general population of around 5%, which means a clearly higher prevalence for pregnant women.

Goodman and co-workers[25] surveyed 500 consecutive pregnant women between 32 and 34 weeks' gestation attending a prenatal clinic in London. When contacted by telephone at 4 weeks postpartum, they found 97 (19%) of the women reporting symptoms consistent with RLS. Thirty percent of the multiparas had experienced RLS in their previous pregnancies, and 16 of 97 had RLS prior to pregnancy, with five reporting exacerbations during the third trimester. The authors stated that those with and without RLS had similar hemoglobin levels and reported similar use of iron and folate supplements. Interestingly, only 26 of 97 women mentioned their RLS symptoms to their healthcare provider.

This powerful analysis underlines the higher prevalence of RLS in pregnancy, but it raises the question: are anemia, low hemoglobin or folate levels the cause of this higher prevalence?

The answer to this question is delivered by Lee and co-workers[26]. They investigated healthy women between 25 and 39 years of age who were planning a pregnancy within the next year. They recruited 45 women planning a pregnancy who were studied during their follicular and luteal phases of the menstrual cycle, and at 11–12 weeks, 23–24 weeks and 35–36 weeks gestation age; 30 women completed the investigation. The prevalence of RLS increased from 0 during preconception to 23% during the third trimester of pregnancy. Only one subject continued to experience RLS after delivery. Compared with those without complaints of RLS, those with RLS had low serum ferritin at preconception and significantly lower folate levels during preconception and at each trimester. In addition, time to sleep onset was significantly delayed and depressed mood was significantly higher in the RLS group. Rather than indicators of iron deficiency anemia (serum ferritin, serum iron and hemoglobin) or pernicious anemia (vitamin B_{12}), it was reduced serum folate level that was associated with RLS in this sample of pregnant women.

In summary, the higher prevalence of RLS during pregnancy seems to be a fact and the reduced folate level in particular during preconception may be a main underlying factor.

NEUROPATHIES AND RADICULOPATHIES

Neuropathies and radiculopathies can co-occur with RLS. O'Hare[27] prospectively determined the prevalence of morbidity from various forms of diabetic neuropathy in a population of 800 patients with diabetes mellitus and in 100 non-diabetic control subjects. The diagnostic criteria for RLS were not quite clear. Whereas 7% of the control population reported RLS, 8.8% of the diabetics were affected. Interestingly, 6.0% of diabetes type I and 10.8% of diabetes type II patients had RLS, indicating a preference for type II diabetics. In accordance with this, Rutkove[28] reports a prevalence of RLS in patients with large- and small-fiber neuropathy of 5–8.8%, rates which were no higher than controls.

However, in 1996 Ondo and Jankovic[16] were able to detect differences in clinical symptomatology between idiopathic and neuropathic patients with RLS. They studied 54 patients who satisfied the diagnostic criteria for RLS. The mean age of the patients was 62.69 years, and the mean age of onset was 34 years. They found that 92% of patients with idiopathic RLS (without neuropathy) had a family history, whereas only 13% of those with neuropathic RLS (associated with peripheral neuropathy) had a positive family history. The sporadic/neuropathic patients were older at symptom onset and tended to have a more rapid progression than the familial/idiopathic patients.

RLS AND PARKINSON'S DISEASE (see also Chapter 6)

The correlation between RLS and Parkinson's disease (PD) has been the focus of several studies. Ondo and colleagues[29] found symptoms of RLS in 20.8% of 303 patients with PD. No controls were used in this study, although the prevalence rate obtained was higher than the one reported in other studies for the elderly, suggesting an association between PD and RLS. Patients with PD and RLS were older, were less likely to have a positive family history for RLS and had lower serum ferritin levels than patients with idiopathic RLS. RLS symptoms in PD appeared to be milder in severity than reported for idiopathic RLS. This observation has been supported by a recent study based in India by Krishnan and associates[18] who reported an occurrence of 7–9% of RLS among PD patients compared with only 0.8% in the Indian controls.

However, not all authors have been able to find a higher prevalence of RLS in PD than in the general population. Thus, Tan and co-workers[31] evaluated 125 consecutive PD outpatients in Singapore, of whom only 0.8% met IRLSSG criteria for RLS. No control groups were used, although the prevalence rate found in PD was not significantly different compared with 0.6% for the Asian population. Thus, RLS prevalence rates in Singapore were not different in PD from those in the general population. Also, Lang and Johnson[32] did not find any RLS symptoms in 100 consecutive PD patients, although two patients reported an inability to remain quiet in the evening or at night.

One study has looked into the prevalence of PD in RLS patients. Thus, Banno and colleagues[33] found extrapyramidal dysfunction in 17% of men and 23% of women, out of a total of 218 RLS patients. Corresponding prevalence in the control (non-RLS) population was 0.2%.

Taken together, most studies suggest an association between PD and RLS. However, the number of studies is still low and any conclusions have to be carefully considered (Table 3.2).

SPINAL ANESTHESIA

Single case reports describe severe restless legs symptoms, as well as periodic limb movements or myoclonic events during[34] and at the end of spinal anesthesia[35–37]. Högl and colleagues[38] carried out a prospective study to investigate these phenomena in detail. Of 161 patients without any history of RLS, 8.7% developed first-onset RLS after spinal anesthesia. The onset of RLS symptoms occurred a mean of 7.3 days after spinal anesthesia. In one patient, new onset RLS symptoms started immediately as the effect of spinal anesthesia was waning; another patient first noticed RLS symptoms 18 days after surgery. Symptoms were transient, with a mean duration of 33 days. None of the patients had a positive family history for RLS and 13 were available for follow-up interviews after a mean of 19.2 months. None of them reported any symptoms suggestive of recurrence of RLS during the period since the previous interview. There was no correlation between post-lumbar puncture headaches and RLS. Post-lumbar headaches occurred in 6.9%. The incidence of spinal anesthesia-associated transitory RLS in this study was thus higher than that of lumbar puncture headache. Low mean corpuscular volume and mean corpuscular hemoglobin were associated with the occurrence of new-onset RLS after spinal anesthesia. No significant correlation was found between hemoglobin, hematocrit, total erythrocyte count, creatinine, urea, or sex, age, position during surgery, pregnancy or

Table 3.2 Epidemiological associates of RLS

Periodic limb movements
Onset in adolescence/childhood
Pregnancy (third trimester)
Iron deficiency anemia
Uremia and end-stage renal failure
Axonal peripheral neuropathy
Parkinson's disease (investigational)

anesthetic agent or dose. Preoperative low MCV and MCH were correlated with postanesthetic RLS in this study, indicating a possibility of iron deficiency as a susceptibility factor[38].

INFLUENCE OF LIFE-STYLE/PREDISPOSING DISEASES

The association of many aspects of life-style or of other diseases with the development of RLS was recently examined. The results of a telephone survey in the continental United States granted by the National Sleep Foundation were published on the internet in 2001 (http://www.sleepfoundation.org/publications/2001poll.html). A total of 1004 telephone interviews were analyzed. Symptoms of RLS were identified in 13% of the sample. The diagnostic criteria for the RLS diagnosis were not stated. Groups that were more likely to experience RLS included: those with household incomes of \$35000 or less (18% vs. 9%), those with lower levels of marital satisfaction (19% vs. 10%), those who rarely or never use the internet (16% vs. 10%), and those with diabetes (29%), arthritis (25%), depression (23%), heart disease (23%), hypertension (21%) and/or night-time heartburn (19%).

In the Kentucky survey, the adjusted odd ratios (95% confidence intervals) for restless legs and diminished general health and poor mental health status were 2.4 (1.4–4.0) and 3.1 (2.0–4.6), respectively. Restless legs were significantly associated with increased age, body mass index, lower income, smoking, lack of exercise, low alcohol consumption and diabetes[3]. Associated factors were also investigated in Ohayon's European study[5] according to three main categories: health variables; consumption of alcohol, coffee, tobacco and medication; and mental disorders. Among the health variables, subjects with musculoskeletal disease were at greater risk of having RLS. Heart disease was significantly higher in RLS. Hypertension (treated or not) was significantly associated with RLS and made an independent significant contribution. Obstructive sleep apnea syndrome and cataplexy were both strong predictors for RLS. Body mass index was a significant independent factor for RLS. Alcohol intake and smoking were more likely in RLS. Users of SSRI medication were also more likely to have RLS. Having a mental disorder had a strong association with RLS.

In the Canadian study based on the general population a special analysis focussing on smoking habits was executed. The estimated risk of a smoker suffering from RLS was not significantly higher. A major limitation of the study is that their measures do not take into account nicotine dose, duration of habit, or degree of dependence[39].

In the study from Ulfberg and associates on 4000 Swedish men, the authors found sleep-related complaints, as well as headache at awakening and daytime headache occurred more frequently among RLS sufferers who also had a tendency toward social isolation. Subjects with RLS more frequently reported depressed mood, reduced libido, hypertension and heart problems. In the parallel study[12] on 200 Swedish women, aged 18–64 years, sleep-related complaints, complaints of daytime headache and social isolation were related to RLS. Subjective problems in performing work due to sleepiness were nine-fold among the women with RLS.

PERIODIC LIMB MOVEMENTS IN SLEEP

Periodic limb movements in sleep (PLMS) were first reported by Lugaresi and colleagues[39] and polysomnographic studies have recorded PLMS (more than five per hour) in up to 87.8% of RLS patients (Figure 3.1). Prevalence estimates of PLMS are variable and range from 6% in the general population to 58% in a sub-population of subjects over 60 years old. PLM can occur in lower and upper limbs during quiet wakefulness as well. The occurrence of RLS and PD remains controversial although two recent

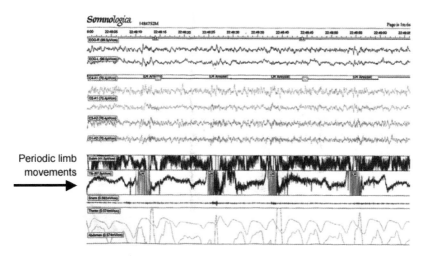

Figure 3.1 Polysomnography profile showing recurrent periodic leg movements during sleep in a RLS patient. Courtesy Dr A Williams, St. Thomas' Hospital, London, UK

observational studies suggest a higher rate of RLS (19.5% and 20%) in patients with PD. However, studies of RLS in PD are limited by methodological problems with the confounding effect of dopaminergic drugs, akathisia, dyskinesias and non-motor symptoms of PD.

CONCLUSIONS

RLS is a common disease in the general population and, since 1995, studies have improved in methodology and surveys in the white Caucasian population suggest that adult prevalence figures of RLS may range from 5% to 15%. Retrospective assessments indicate that onset of RLS may occur before the age of 20 years in up to 43% of adult cases. There are no prevalence data related to RLS available from the UK. Based on current estimates, there may be 8–10 million sufferers in the UK alone.

RLS may be associated with iron deficiency anemia, renal failure/uremia, pregnancy and, possibly, PD. A single study by Mathews[40] suggested that 43% of patients with iron deficiency may have 'leg restlessness', while several studies report a 20% to 57% prevalence of RLS in renal dialysis patients. Reports of RLS in patients with large and small fiber neuropathy are variable and range from 5% to 8.8%, rates not higher than controls. During pregnancy, RLS has been reported in 11–27% of women, usually during the third trimester.

REFERENCES

1. Ekbom KA. Restless legs syndrome. *Neurology* 1960;10:868–73

2. Walters AS. International Restless Legs Syndrome Study Group. Towards a better definition of restless legs syndrome. *Mov Disord* 1995;10:634–42

3. Phillips B, Young T, Finn L, *et al*. Epidemiology of restless legs symptoms in adults. *Arch Intern Med* 2000;160:2137–41

4. Lavigne GJ, Montplaisir JY. Restless legs syndrome and sleep bruxism: prevalence and association among Canadians. *Sleep* 1994;17:739–43

5. Ohayon M, Roth T. Prevalence of restless legs syndrome and periodic limb movements disorder in the general population. *J Psychosom Res* 2002;53: 547–54

6. Ulfberg J, Nyström B, Carter N, Edling C. Restless legs syndrome among men aged 18 to 64 years: An association with somatic disease and neuropsychiatric symptoms. *Mov Disord* 2001;16:1159–63

7. Rothdach AJ, Trenkwalder C, Haberstock J, *et al*. Prevalence and risk factors of RLS in an elderly population. The MEMO study. *Neurology* 2000;54:1064–8

8. Montplaisir J, Boucher S, Poirier G, *et al*. Clinical, polysomnographic, and genetic characteristics of restless legs syndrome: a study of 133 patients diagnosed with the new standard criteria. *Mov Disord* 1997;12:61–5

9. Walters AS, Picchietti D, Hening W, Lazzarini A. Variable expressivity in familial restless legs syndrome. *Neurology* 1994;44:A217–18

10. Walters AS, Hickey K, Maltzmann J, *et al*. A questionnaire study of 138 patients with restless legs syndrome: The 'Night-Walkers' survey. *Neurology* 1996;46:92–5

12. Ulfberg J, Nyström B, Carter N, Edling C. Restless legs syndrome among working-aged women. *Eur Neurol* 2001a;46:17–19

13. Ekbom KA. Astenia crurum paraesthetica (irritable legs). *Acta Med Scand* 1944;118:197

14. Winkelmann J, Wetter TC, Collado-Seidel V, *et al*. Clinical characteristics and frequency of the hereditary restless legs syndrome in a population of 300 patients. *Sleep* 2000;23:597–602

15. Godbout R, Montplaisir J, Poirier G. Epidemiological data in familial restless legs syndrome. *Sleep Res* 1987;16:338

16. Ondo W, Jankovic J. Restless legs syndrome: clinicoetiologic correlates. *Neurology* 1996;47:1435–41

17. Tan EK, Seah A, See SJ, *et al*. Restless legs syndrome in an Asian population: A study in Singapore. *Mov Disord* 2001;16:577–9

18. Krishnan PR, Bhatia M, Behar M. Restless legs syndrome in Parkinson's disease: a case controlled study. *Mov Disord* 2003;18:181–5

19. Callaghan N. Restless legs in uremic neuropathy. *Neurology* 1996;16:359–61

20. Rogers SD, Harris DCH, Stewart JH. Possible relation between restless legs and anaemia in renal dialysis patients. *Lancet* 1991;337:1551

21. Winkelmann JW, Chertow GM, Lazarus JM. Restless legs syndrome in end-stage renal disease. *Am J Kidney Dis* 1996;28:372–8

22. Yasuda T, Nishimura A, Katsuki Y, Tsuji Y. Restless legs syndrome treated successfully by kidney transplantation—a case report. *Clin Transpl* 1986:138

23. Nordlander NB. Therapy in restless legs. *Acta Med Scand* 1953;145:453–7

24. O'Keefe ST, Gavin K, Lavan N. Iron status and restless legs syndrome in the elderly. *Age Ageing* 1994;23:200–3

25. Goodman JDS, Brodie C, Ayida GA. Restless legs syndrome in pregnancy. *Br Med J* 1988;297:1101

26. Lee KA, Zaffke ME, Baratte-Beebe K. Restless legs syndrome and sleep disturbance during pregnancy: the role of folate and iron. *J Womens Health* 2001;10:335–41

27. O'Hare JA, Abuaisha F, Geoghegan M. Prevalence and forms of neuropathic morbidity in 800 diabetics. *Ir J Med Sci* 1994;163:132–5

28. Rutkove SB, Matheson JK, Logigian EL. Restless legs syndrome in patients with polyneuropathy. *Muscle Nerve* 1996;19:670–2

29. Ondo WG, Vuong KD, Jankovic J. Exploring the relationship between Parkinson's disease and restless legs syndrome. *Arch Neurol* 2002;59:421–4

30. Krishnan PR, Bhatia M, Behari M. Restless legs syndrome in Parkinson's disease: A case controlled study. *Mov Disord* 2003;18:181–5

31. Tan EK, Lum SY, Wong MC. Restless legs syndrome in Parkinson's disease. *J Neurol Sci* 2002;196:33–6

32. Lang AE, Johnson K. Akathisia in idiopathic Parkinson´s disease. *Neurology* 1987;37:477–81

33. Banno K, Delaive K, Walld R, Kryger MH. Restless legs syndrome in 218 patients: associated disorders. *Sleep Med* 2000;1:221–9

34. Watanabe S, Sakai K, Ono Y, *et al*. Alternating periodic leg movement induced by spinal anesthesia in an elderly male. *Anesth Analg* 1987;66:1031–2

35. Lee MS, Lyoo CH, Kim WC, Kang HJ. Periodic bursts of rhythmic dyskinesia associated with spinal anesthesia. *Mov Disord* 1997;12:816–17

36. Fox EJ, Villanueva R, Schutta HS. Myoclonus following spinal anesthesia. *Neurology* 1979;29:379–80

37. Nadkarni AV, Tondare AS. Localized clonic convulsions after spinal anesthesia with lidocaine and epinephrine. *Anesth Analg* 1982;61:945–7

38. Högl B, Frauscher B, Seppi K, *et al*. Transient restless legs syndrome after spinal anesthesia. A prospective study. *Neurology* 2002;59:1705–7

39. Lavigne GJ, Lobbezoo F, Rompre PH, *et al*. Cigarette smoking as a risk factor or an exacerbating factor for restless legs syndrome and sleep bruxism. *Sleep* 2001;20:290–3

40. Matthews WB. Iron deficiency and restless legs [Letter]. *Br Med J* 1976;1:898

41. Lugaresi E, Coccagna G, Mantovani M, Lebrun R. Some periodic phenoma arising during drowsiness and sleep in man. *Electroencephalogr Clin Neurophysiol* 1972;32:701–5

4 Pathophysiology of restless legs syndrome

M. Mrowka, K. Ray Chaudhuri and P. Odin

The pathophysiology of restless legs syndrome (RLS) remains unknown. Originally, the peripheral location of the symptoms suggested a peripheral origin of RLS, but the results of research in recent years point towards a central nervous system dysfunction. It is likely that RLS occurs from a complex interaction of peripheral and central nervous system factors. A range of pharmacologic, neurophysiologic, circadian, genetic and functional imaging studies have contributed to an improved understanding of the pathophysiology of RLS.

PHARMACOLOGIC BASIS OF RLS

Low-dose intake of levodopa or an opioid often leads to relief from symptoms of RLS[1–5]. Moreover, not only dopamine precursors, but also dopamine agonists improve RLS symptoms according to a number of studies evaluating treatment of RLS[6–10]. Similarly, centrally active dopamine antagonists, such as neuroleptics, tricyclic antidepressive drugs and caffeine, cause a worsening of the RLS symptoms, whereas RLS is not worsened by peripherally active dopaminergic antagonists such as domperidone.

The opioid system is also likely to be involved in the genesis of RLS. This was noted by Willis[14] in the 17th century, while Ekbom in 1945[15] described a positive effect from opioids on the symptoms of RLS. In patients with RLS the dopamine receptor antagonist pimozide could neutralize the positive effect from the opioid receptor agonist codeine[16]. On the other hand it was not possible to inhibit the effect of the dopamine agonist bromocriptine with the opioid antagonist naloxone. In another study naloxone could exacerbate RLS symptoms in patients with opioid premedication[17], whereas opioid antagonists did not provoke symptoms in untreated patients[18]. All these results demonstrate that the dopaminergic and the opioid systems can play important roles in the pathophysiology of RLS, although it is still unclear how the two systems interact in these functions.

Currently the first-line treatment of RLS is with dopaminergic agents. However, in contrast to the treatment of patients with Parkinson's disease, there appears to be no sign of development of motor fluctuations or dyskinesias in RLS, although with levodopa and some dopamine agonists augmentation[19] may occur in RLS patients. This differential reaction to dopaminergic treatment indicates that the involvement of the dopaminergic system in RLS is dissimilar to nigrostriatal denervation as seen in Parkinson's disease.

FUNCTIONAL IMAGING STUDIES

In order to investigate the involvement of the dopaminergic system in RLS, a number of functional imaging studies with single photon emission computer tomography (SPECT), as well as positron emission tomography (PET) techniques, have been performed. These studies have shown variable and inconsistent results. Reduction of presynaptic dopaminergic function has been found in two studies in RLS patients using ^{18}F-dopa; Ruottinen and co-workers[20] reported a slight decrease of uptake of 12% in the caudate and 11% in the putamen, and Turjanski and colleagues[21] reported a modest but significant decrease in the putamen, but not in the caudate nucleus[20,21]. On the other hand, Michaud and associates[22] found no significant pathology in ten patients investigated with beta-CIT-SPECT. Trenkwalder and co-workers[23] could not confirm impaired ^{18}F-dopa uptake in the striatum in a small group of four patients. Eisensehr and colleagues[24] used IPT-SPECT and found no presynaptic differences in 14 drug-naïve and 11 levodopa-treated patients with RLS in comparison with age-matched normal controls. Mrowka and associates[25] also have been unable to confirm any significant changes in presynaptic dopamine transporter binding, but a relatively altered uptake of ^{123}I-beta-CIT in putamen versus the caudate nucleus was found. In the latter study, mild hypokinesia and rigidity were found in a subgroup of RLS patients, when examined with clinical testing and computerized movement analysis. These symptoms improved with levodopa, further supporting a dopaminergic involvement[10,25].

Focusing on the postsynaptic side of the dopaminergic system, Turjanski[21] showed a decreased binding potential of D_2 receptors with raclopride-PET, and two studies showed a lower postsynaptic striatal D_2 binding in ^{123}IBZM-SPECT in patients with nocturnal myoclonus syndrome, as well as in patients with RLS[22,26]. Eisensehr and co-workers[24] could not, however, demonstrate any postsynaptic pathology with IBZM-SPECT in 14 drug-naïve and 11 levodopa-treated patients with RLS.

There could be several reasons for the discrepancy in these results: in some studies there was a significant age difference between RLS patients and controls and the concentration of D_2 receptors shows an age dependence with decline in age. In addition, all studies so far ignore the fact that the clinical symptoms of patients with RLS are most pronounced in the evening or at night. Hypothetically, the pathology in the dopaminergic system might be transient and better detectable in the evening or night. Furthermore, the investigations so far have focused on the nigrostriatal dopaminergic system, whereas the pathology of RLS may be located in the diencephalospinal or the mesolimbic dopaminergic system. Therefore, imaging studies involving other ligands, performed at timepoints such as night-time, would be of interest.

Evidence supporting a subcortical site as a location for the dysfunction in RLS is suggested by magnetic resonance imaging (MRI) studies. Whereas no structural abnormalities were noted in MRI studies[27], functional MRI showed bilateral activation of the cerebellum and contralateral activation of thalamus during sensory symptoms (without movements), and in the pons and red nucleus when these sensory events were accompanied by movements.

CIRCADIAN RHYTHMIC OF RLS AND METABOLIC SYSTEMS

A key feature of RLS is its diurnal variation and, as dopamine has influence on the secretion of prolactin and growth hormone, Wetter and co-workers[28] examined the level of these hormones over 24 hours and compared them with those of a normal healthy control population. They found no significant differences between the groups. This indicates that the dopaminergic dysfunction is unlikely to have an influence on the endocrine rhythms in RLS.

Considering that the iron metabolism has a circadian rhythmic too, with a high level of serum iron at midday and a decreased level at midnight[29,30], together with the fact that iron deficiency anemia is associated with RLS, another research focus has been on examinations of the role of the iron in the pathophysiology of RLS[31]. Ekbom himself described iron deficiency in 25% of patients with RLS, suggested that the lack of iron is a reason for the high incidence of RLS in pregnancy, and treated patients with iron substitution[32]. The possible role of iron is emphasized by the negative correlation between the level of ferritin and the severity of the RLS symptoms[33]. Studies on cerebrospinal fluid (CSF) showed a decreased ferritin and elevated transferrin in patients with RLS in comparison with healthy persons[31]. An MRI study in five patients with RLS demonstrated a decreased iron concentration in the putamen and in the substantia nigra in patients with RLS[34]. As iron is a co-factor for the dopamine-producing enzyme thyrosine hydroxylase, there is a possible link between iron deficit and a dopaminergic deficit. Lower dopamine concentrations could be the result of low iron levels. Moreover, iron is important for the functioning of dopamine D_2 receptors, so that iron deficiency could also induce an impairment of the normal receptor function[35].

PARKINSON'S DISEASE AND RLS

Few studies have systematically addressed the issue of RLS occurring in Parkinson's disease (PD). This issue is compounded by the fact that RLS is often treated by dopaminergic drugs and symptoms of RLS may overlap with akathisia and nocturnal motor fluctuations. A study by Ondo and colleagues[36] surveyed 320 patients and analyzed records of 303 PD patents. They reported RLS in 19.5% of the PD patients. Arnulf and co-workers[37] have suggested that routine polysomnography and MSLT evaluation in PD would unmask PLM in 15% of cases. Increased PLM index has also been reported in untreated PD patients. Further studies investigating the relationship of PD and RLS are thus required. The dopaminergic basis of RLS is also supported by the often dramatic response of RLS to dopaminergic drugs such as levodopa or dopamine agonists and by recent reports of amelioration of RLS and PLM in PD following pallidotomy. Recently a family, family LA with RLS and parkin gene mutation (8 out of 17 patients), some of whom developed signs of PD have been described[38].

Genetics

Between 42% and 90% of RLS patients have RLS in the family[39–42]. The mode of inheritance seems to be autosomal-dominant with a high penetrance[43,44]. The degree of expression of RLS symptoms varies within the families[45]. It seems that hereditary RLS starts at an earlier age compared with the sporadic form. In some cases there have also been signs of anticipation; thus it appears that the disease starts earlier with each new generation[43].

In order to examine the genetic substrate of the dopaminergic hypothesis in RLS, Desautels and co-workers[46] have analyzed eight genes coding for receptors and enzymes related to dopaminergic transmission, using a population of 92 patients with RLS and 182 controls. The results suggested that the chosen loci have no major effect on vulnerability to RLS. Moreover, stratification analyses according to age at onset and PLMS index disclosed no significant differences for any of the polymorphisms examined. These findings, however, do not rule out an involvement of the dopaminergic system in RLS symptomatology and continued genetic studies are highly warranted.

Recently, three loci showing vulnerability to RLS have been descibed in French-Canadian and Italian families in chromosomes 12q, 14q and 9q[47–49]. None of these loci are clearly related to the dopaminergic system. Desautels and co-workers[47] reported the first identification of a susceptibility locus for RLS on chromosome 12q in a French-Canadian family. The genes involved may be the timeless gene or the gene encoding neurotensin, a neuropeptide thought to be a neuromodulator of dopaminergic neurotransmission. However, the true mode of inheritance in this family is autosomal recessive. Bonati and colleagues[48] have reported significant evidence of linkage to a new locus for RLS on chromosome 14q13–21 region in a 30-member, three-generation Italian family affected by RLS and periodic leg movements in sleep (PLMS). This is the first RLS locus consistent with an autosomal dominant inheritance pattern. More recently, Chen *et al.* have performed genome-wide linkage scan to identify a novel susceptibility locus for RLS on chromosome 9p24-22 based on 144 subjects[49].

SPINAL CORD AND RLS

A dysfunction of other dopamine-dependent pathways, such as the diencephalospinal pathway, has been suggested as an alternative mechanism for RLS. It is possible that the spinal cord could be involved in the generation of periodic leg movements (PLM), since RLS symptoms and PLM have been observed in connection with spinal cord lesions and illnesses[50–59]. Also, transient RLS symptoms can appear after spinal anesthesia[60]. It has thus been suggested that PLM arise from a loss of supraspinal inhibitory impulses, resulting in enhanced facilitation of spinal flexor reflexes. The fact that PLM occur also after complete spinal interruption suggests that the primary generator for PLM is likely to be spinal. However, treatment with levodopa causes only a mild reduction of the rate of PLM after spinal cord injury compared with a very marked improvement seen in RLS[61]. Also, the fact that there are differences in the nature of the PLM[59] and in the circadian and sleep regulation of PLM indicates that the mechanisms behind PLM in RLS and spinal cord lesions, respectively, might partly differ.

NEUROPHYSIOLOGIC STUDIES

In an early study on PLM, Smith and co-workers[62] found that they have similarities with the Babinsky reflex. As a less pronounced Babinsky-like movement also normally occurs in non-REM sleep, the authors postulated that PLM could be an effect of reduced supraspinal inhibitory mechanisms. Studies on cortical activity have so far not proved a cortical involvement for RLS. Thus, no cortical pre-potentials have been observed in association with either RLS or PLMS[18,63]. However, the response to paired transcranial magnetic stimulation suggested reduced intracortical inhibition for both feet and hand muscles[64]. Two further studies indicated reduced supraspinal inhibition in RLS patients[65,66], thus suggesting a subcortical dysfunction altering the motor pathways. After administration of levodopa the supraspinal inhibition was nearly normalized in patients with RLS[66]. It is, however, not clear if this inhibitory effect of levodopa takes place at a spinal, basal ganglial or cortical level.

Brain-stem reflex studies have so far failed to show abnormal CNS function in RLS. In general, brain-stem and transcortical studies have been found to be normal[67,68]. This speaks against structural damage at the brain-stem level. However, a recent study showed an abnormal modulation of the spinal flexor response as measured by stimulation of the medial plantar nerve and bilateral recording from antagonist leg and thigh muscles. A state-dependent increased excitability was found during sleep in ten RLS patients compared with wakefulness or controls, suggesting a reversal in RLS of the normal sleep- or circadian-related spinal cord inhibition, thus causing an increased spinal cord excitability[69]. The fact that dopaminergic substances influence the excitability of the flexor reflex[70] enhances the role of dopaminergic systems in the pathophysiology.

The role of the peripheral nervous system in RLS is still unclear. RLS symptoms have been described in connection with different types of polyneuropathy, and recently in Charcot–Marie–Tooth types I and II[71]. Sural nerve biopsies from patients with idiopathic RLS have shown abnormalities and also the response to temperature stimulation has been reported to be abnormal. This can indicate that RLS patients have a subclinical axonal neuropathy. Whether the peripheral changes have a primary or rather a secondary role in the pathophysiology is, however, unclear.

RECENT ADVANCES

Pioneering work using tissue from brains of RLS patients and controls from Allen and colleagues in USA have recently reported that transferrin receptor expression by neuromelanin cells are decreased in RLS[73]. This work follows from their earlier report that in RLS, there is impaired brain iron acquisition[74] and strengthens the hypothesis that RLS, at least in part, may arise from a central cellular iron deficiency caused by a defect in iron regulatory protein-1 in neuromelanin cells of the brain. An inbred strain of mice which expresses low iron in ventral midbrain and high liver iron have recently been developed by the same group as a possible animal model of RLS which may aid behavioural, neurochemical and genetic analysis[75].

CONCLUSION

In summary, RLS seems to involve disturbances in the central dopaminergic system, iron metabolism and opioid neurotransmission, but the details of these disturbances largely remain to be explored (Figure 4.1). The

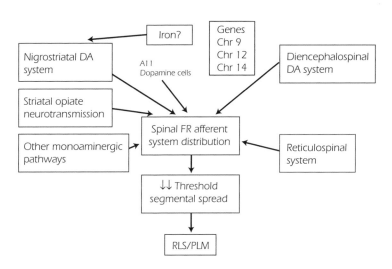

Figure 4.1 Possible pathophysiologic basis of restless legs syndrome (RLS) and periodic limb movements (PLM). DA, dopaminergic; FR, flexor reflex. Iron metabolism and genetic influences are likely to be important. Striatal opiate system abnormalities may be important. From Chaudhuri KR[20]

changes in the dopaminergic system, seem to be relatively discrete, and may fluctuate with time. Other brain areas than the nigrostriatal dopaminergic system seem to play an important role. Recent evidence suggests that the iron metabolic system and intracellular iron in addition to the opioid neurotransmission system may play a key role in pathogenesis of RLS. Also, RLS symptomatology seems to depend on abnormal sensorimotor integration, supernormal excitability at the spinal level and probably reduced supraspinal inhibitory mechanisms. Further neurophysiologic–neuropharmacologic, neuropathologic and neurogenetic studies may help with the clarification of the pathophysiology behind RLS.

REFERENCES

1. Hening W, Allen R, Earley C, *et al*. The treatment of restless legs syndrome and periodic limb movement disorder – an American Academy of Sleep Medicine Review. *Sleep* 1999;22:970–98

2. Acpinar S. Treatment of restless legs syndrome with levodopa plus benserazide. *Arch Neurol* 1982;39:739

3. Montplaisir J, Godbout R, Poirier G, Bedard MA. Restless legs syndrome and periodic movements in sleep: physiopathology and treatment with L-dopa. *Clin Neuropharmacol* 1986;9:456–63

4. Walters AS, Wagner ML, Hening WA, *et al*. Succesful treatment of the idiopathic restless legs syndrome in a randomized double-blind trial of ocycodone versus placebo. *Sleep* 1993;16:327–32

5. Akpinar S. Restless legs syndrome treatment with dopaminergic drugs. *Clin Neuropharmacol* 1987:10:69–79

6. Stiasny K, Roebbecke J, Schüler P, Oertel WH. The treatment of idiopathic restless legs syndrome (RLS) with the D2-agonist cabergoline – an open clinical trial. *Sleep* 2000;23:349–54

7. Montplaisir J, Denesle R, Petit D. Pramipexole in the treatment of restless legs syndrome – a follow-up study. *Eur J Neurol* 2000;7:27–31

8. Stiasny K. Clinical data on restless legs syndrome: a dose finding study with cabergoline. *Eur J Neurol* 2001;46:24–6

9. Ondo W. Ropinirole for restless legs syndrome. *Mov Disord* 1999;14:138–40

10. Odin P, Mrowka M, Shing M. Restless legs syndrome. *Eur J Neurol* 2002;9:1–9

11. Wetter TC, Stiasny K, Winkelmann J, *et al*. A randomized controlled study of pergolide in patients with restless legs syndrome. *Neurology* 1999;52:944–50

12. Winkelmann J, Schadrack J, Wetter TC, Zieglgängsberger W, Trenkwalder C. Opioid and dopamine antagonist drug challenges in untreated restless legs syndrome patients. *Sleep Med* 2001;2:57–61

13. Kraus T, Schuld A, Pollmächer T. Periodic leg movements in sleep and restless legs syndrome probably caused by olanzapine. *Clin Psychopharmacol* 1999;19:478–9

14. Willis T. *The London Practice of Physick*. T. London: Bassett Crooke, 1685:404

15. Ekbom KA. Restless legs syndrome. *Acta Med Scand* 1945;158:4–122

16. Montplaisir J, Lorrain D, Godbout R. Restless legs syndrome and periodic movements in sleep: the primary role of dopaminergic mechanism. *Eur Neurol* 1991:31;411–43

17. Walters AS, Hening W. Review of the clinical presentation and neuropharmacology of the restless legs syndrome. *Clin Neuropharmacol* 1987;10:225–37

18. Lugaresi E, Cirignotta F, Coccagna G, Montagna P. *Myoclonus. Advances in Neurology*. New York: Raven Press, 1986

19. Allen RP, Earley CJ. Augmentation of the restless legs syndrome with carbidopa/levodopa. *Sleep* 1996;19: 205–13

20. Ruottinen HM, Partinen M, Hublin C, *et al*. A FDOPA PET study in patients with periodic limb movement disorder and restless legs sydnrom. *Neurology* 2000;54:502–4

21. Turjanski N, Lees AJ, Brooks DJ. Striatal dopaminergic function in restless legs syndrome: ^{18}F-dopa and ^{11}C-raclopride PET studies. *Neurology* 1999;52:932–7

22. Michaud M, Sourcy J-P, Chabli A, *et al*. SPECT imaging of striatal pre- and postsynaptic dopaminergic status in restless legs syndrome with periodic leg movements in sleep. *J Neurol* 2002;249:164–70

23. Trenkwalder C, Walters AS, Hening WA, *et al*. Positron emission tomographic studies in restless legs syndrome. *Mov Disord* 1999:14;141–5

24. Eisensehr I, Wetter TC, Linke R, *et al*. Normal IPT and IBZM SPECT in drug-naive and levodopa-treated idiopathic restless legs syndrome. *Neurology* 2001;57:1307–9

25. Mrowka M, Joebges M, Berding G, *et al*. Clinical investigations, computerized movement analysis and striatal dopamine transporter function in restless legs syndrome. *J Neural Transm* 2001;108:P120

26. Staedt J, Stoppe G, Koegler A, *et al*. Nocturnal myoclonus syndrome (periodic movements in sleep) related to central dopamine D_2-receptor alteration. *Eur Arch Psychiatry Clin Neurosci* 1995:245:8–10

27. Bucher SF, Seelos KC, Oertel WH, *et al*. Cerebral generators involved in the pathogenesis of the restless legs syndrome. *Ann Neurol* 1997;41:639–45

28. Wetter TC, Collado-Seidel V, Oertel H, *et al*. Endocrine rhythms in patients with restless legs syndrome. *J Neurol* 2002;249:146–51

29. Scales WE, Vander AJ, Brown MB, Kluger MJ. Human circadian rhythms in temperature, trace metals, and blood variables. *J Appl Physiol* 1988;65:1840–6

30. Tarquini B. Iron metabolism: clinical chronobiological aspects. *Chronobiologica* 1978;5:315–6

31. Earley CJ, Allen RP, Beard JL, Conner JR. Insight into the pathophysiology of restless legs syndrome. *J Neurosci Res* 2000;62:623–8

32. Ekbom A. Restless legs syndrome. *Neurology* 1960;10:868–73

33. O'Keefe ST, Gavin K, Lavan JN. Iron status and restless legs syndrome in the elderly. *Age Ageing* 1994;23:200–3

34. Allen RP, Baker PB, Wehrl F, *et al.* MRI measurement of brain iron in patients with restless legs syndrome. *Neurology* 2001;56:263–5

35. Chokroverty S, Jankovic J. Restless legs syndrome. *Neurology* 1999;52:907

36. Ondo WG, Vuong KD, Atassi F, *et al.* Daytime sleepiness and other sleep disorders in Parkinson's disease. *Neurology* 2001;57:1392–6

37. Arnulf I, Konofal E, Merino-Andreu M, *et al.* Parkinson's disease and sleepiness: an integral part of PD. *Neurology* 2002;58:1019–24

38. Maniak S, Kabakei K, Pichler I, Kramer PL, Pramstaller C. Restless legs syndrome (RLS) in a large family (Family LA) with *Parkin*-associated Parkinson's disease (PD). *Mov Disord* 2004;19 (Suppl 9):S354

39. Montplaisir J, Boucher S, Poirier G, *et al.* Clinical, polysomnographic, and genetic characteristics of restless legs syndrome: a study of 133 patients diagnosed with new standard criteria. *Mov Disord* 1997;12:61–5

40. Ondo W, Jankovic J. Restless legs syndrome: clinicoetiologic correlates. *Neurology* 1996;47:1435–41

41. Walters AS, Hickey K, Maltzman J, *et al.* A questionnaire study of 138 patients with restless legs syndrome: the 'Night-Walkers' survey. *Neurology* 1996;46:92–5

42. Winkelmann J, Wetter TC, Collado-Seidel V, *et al.* Clinical characteristics and frequency of the hereditary restless legs syndrome in a population of 300 patients. *Sleep* 2000;23:597–602

43. Lazzarini A, Walters AS, Hickey K, *et al.* Studies of penetrance and anticipation in five autosomal-dominant restless legs syndrome pedigrees. *Mov Disord* 1999;14:111–16

44. Winkelmann J, Muller-Myhsok B, Wittchen HU, *et al.* Complex segregation analysis of restless legs syndrome provides evidence for an autosomal dominant mode of inheritance in early age at onset families. *Ann Neurol* 2002;52:297–302

45. Walters AS, Picchietti D, Hening W, Lazzarini A. Variable expressivity in familial restless legs syndrome. *Arch Neurol* 1990;47:1219–20

46. Desautels A, Turecki G, Montplaisir J, *et al.* Dopaminergic neurotransmission and restless legs syndrome: a genetic association analysis. *Neurology* 2001;57:1304–6

47. Desautels A, Turecki G, Montplaisir J, *et al.* Evidence for a genetic association between monoamine oxidase A and restless legs syndrome. *Neurology* 2002;59:215–19

48. Bonati MT, Ferini-Strambi L, Aridon P, *et al.* Autosomal dominant restless legs syndrome maps on chromosome 14q. *Brain* 2003;126:1485–92

49. Chen S, Ondo W, Rao S, Li L, Chen Q, Wang Q. Genomewide linkage scan identifies a novel susceptibility locus for restless legs syndrome on chromosome 9p. *Am J Hum Genet* 2004;74:876–85

50. Abele M, Buerk K, Laccone F, *et al*. Restless legs syndrome in Spinocerebellar ataxia Types 1, 2 and 3. *J Neurol* 2001;248:311–14

51. Dickel MJ, Renfrow SD, Moore PT, Berry RB. Rapid eye movement sleep periodic leg movements in patients with spinal cord injury. *Sleep* 1994; 17: 733–8

52. Hartmann M, Pfister R, Pfadenhauer K. Restless legs syndrome associated with spinal cord lesions. *J Neurol Neurosurg Psychiatry* 1999;66:688–97

53. Hemmer B, Riemann D, Glocker FX, *et al*. Restless legs syndrome after Borrelia-induced myelitis. *Mov Disord* 1995;10:521–6

54. Lee M, Choi YC, Lee SH, Lee SB. Sleep-related periodic leg movements associated with spinal cord lesions. *Mov Disord* 1996;11:719–22

55. De Mello MT, Lauro FA, Silva AC, Tufik S. Incidence of periodic leg movements and of the restless legs syndrome during sleep following acute physical activity in spinal cord injury subjects. *Spinal Cord* 1996;34:294–6

56. Nogues M, Cammarota A, Leiguarda R, *et al*. Periodic limb movements in syringomyelia and syringobulbia. *Mov Disord* 2000;15:113–19

57. Ondo W, Jankovic J. Restless legs syndrome: clinicoetiologic correlates. *Neurology* 1996;47:1435–41

58. Winkelmann J, Trenkwalder C. Pathophysiology of restless-legs syndrome. Review of current research. *Nervenarzt* 2001;72:100–7

59. Yokota T, Hirose K, Tanabe H, Tsukagoshi H. Sleep-related periodic leg movements (nocturnal myoclonus) due to spinal cord lesion. *J Neurol Sci* 1991;104:13–18

60. Hogl B, Frauscher B, Seppi K, *et al*. Transient restless legs syndrome after spinal anesthesia: a prospective study. *Neurology* 2002;59:1705–7

61. Kaplan PW, Allen RP, Buchholz DW, Walters JK. A double-blind, placebo-controlled study of the treatment of periodic limb movements in sleep using carbidopa/levodopa and propoxyphene. *Sleep* 1993;16:717–23

62. Smith RC. Relationship of periodic movements in sleep (nocturnal myoclonus) and the Babinski sign. *Sleep* 1985;8:239–43

63. Trenkwalder C, Bucher SF, Oertel WH, *et al*. Bereitschaftspotential in idiopathic and symptomatic restless legs syndrome. *Electroencephalogr Clin Neurophysiol* 1993;89:95–103

64. Tergau F, Wischer S, Paulus W. Motor system exitability in patients with restless legs syndrome. *Neurology* 1999;52:1060–3

65. Entezari-Taher M, Singleton JR, Jones CR, *et al*. Changes in excitability of motor circuitry in primary restless legs syndrome. *Neurology* 1999;53:1201–5

66. Stiasny K, Haeske H, Mueller HH, *et al*. Impairment of cortical inhibition in restless legs syndrome—shortening of silent period induced by transcranial magnetic stimulation. *Sleep* 2000;23:A128

67. Bucher SF, Trenkwalder C, Oertel WH. Reflex studies and MRI in restless legs syndrome. *Acta Neurol Scand* 1996;94:145–50

68. Mosko SS, Nudleman KL. Somatosensory and brainstem auditory evoked responses in sleep-related periodic leg movements. *Sleep* 1986;9:399–404

69. Bara-Jimenez W, Aksu M, Graham B, *et al*. Periodoc limb movements in sleep: state-dependent excitability of the spinal flexor reflex. *Neurology* 2000;54: 1609–16

70. Schomburg ED, Steffens H. Comparative analysis of L-DOPA actions on nociceptive and non-nociceptive spinal reflex pathways in the cat. *Neurosci Res* 1998;31:307–16

71. Iannaccones S, Zucconi M, Marchettini P. Evidence of peripheral axonal neuropathy in primary restless legs syndrome. *Mov Disord* 1995;10:2–9

72. Chaudhuri KR. The restless legs syndrome: time to recognize a common movement disorder. *Fract Neurol* 2003;3:204–13

73. Connor JR, Boyer PJ, Menzies J, *et al*. Neuropathological examination suggests impaired brain iron acquisition in restless legs syndrome. *Neurology* 2003;61:304–309

74. Connor JR, Wang XS, Patton SM, Menzies SL, Troncoso JC, Earley CJ, Allen RP. Decreased transferring receptor expression by neuromelanin celss in restless legs syndrome. *Neurology* 2004;62:1563–1567

75. Jones BC, Chesler EJ, Williams RW, Beard JL, Allen RP, Earley CJ. An inbredstrain of mice as an animal model of restless legs syndrome (RLS). *Mov Disord* 2004;19 (Suppl 9):S421

5   Clinical features

C. Meilak, V. Dhawan and K. Ray Chaudhuri

The diagnosis of restless legs syndrome (RLS) is made clinically and clinicians need to identify the key symptoms, as shown in Table 5.1. As discussed before, these symptoms form the minimal criteria which have been universally accepted for the diagnosis of RLS since 1995.

The commonest complaint is usually that of sensory symptoms, principally in the lower limbs associated with a compulsion to move the legs, which offers some relief[1-6]. Sleep disruption is a salient feature, as symptoms are worse at rest or when lying down at night. Sometimes the discomfort is relieved by movement and also by voluntary actions such as rubbing the limbs, but such actions may disrupt sleep further.

It is possible for the entire lower limbs to be affected, but more commonly the area between the ankle and the knee is where the problem lies. The urge to move the limbs is most frequent in the legs but a similar sensation may also occur in the upper limbs, and in one series of patients with idiopathic RLS, 48.7% reported upper limb restlessness. This may be misleading in diagnosis, so an awareness of how commonly by these additional arm symptoms occur is important.

Clinically the sensory aspect of RLS can be divided into the classical (sensory) or pain-dominated symptoms. This distinction was originally recognized by Ekbom[7].

Patients often use a variety of ways to describe these sensations and it is likely that the descriptions (some listed in Table 5.2) vary according to

Table 5.1   Criteria for the diagnosis of idiopathic RLS

1.	The four main criteria of RLS
2.	The need to move limbs, often associated with abnormal sensations such as dysesthesia
3	Motor restlessness
4.	Symptoms are usually worse or only present when at rest. Movement provides momentary relief
5.	Symptoms are worse in the evening or at night

culture, local beliefs and expressions. For some, it is a clear description of pain; others describe generalized discomfort and cramps which may be caused by a condition other than RLS.

Other features that commonly occur in RLS and which are associated with the disease are summarized in Table 5.3. However, the presence of these additional features is not mandatory for diagnosis. Sleep disturbance commonly occurs, especially during initiating sleep, which then leads to daytime somnolence, a prominent complaint of the RLS sufferer which impacts greatly on quality of life. However, profound daytime sleepiness is uncommon in RLS[1-5].

Another characteristic commonly associated with RLS is periodic limb movements in sleep (PLMS) or while awake (PMLW), described as repetitive flexing of the lower limb joints (hip, knee or ankle, occasionally the upper limb) and the dorsiflexion or fanning of the toes[8]. This characteristic may become apparent on questioning sufferer's partner as his/her sleep may also be disturbed. The usual frequency of these limb movements is every 5–90 seconds and lasting from 0.5 to 5 seconds each. The etiology of PLMS may

Table 5.2   Descriptions by patients of RLS sensations in the legs

Pins and needles	Itching bones
Aching calves	Electric shocks
Like having a toothache in the legs	Legs tearing open
Throbbing pain	Cold water down legs
Leg cramps	Burning in legs
Creepy-crawly sensation	'Elvis legs'
Pulling feeling	

Table 5.3   Additional features of RLS

Insomnia
Involuntary movements – PLMS, PLMW
Positive family history
Chronic progressive course ± periodic exacerbations
Normal neurologic examination (except possible neuropathy)
Responsive to dopaminergic drugs

involve a central or peripheral dopaminergic hypothesis and the risk of developing this may increase with age. These movements are different from leg/body jerks that can occur while falling asleep, the so-called 'hypnic jerks'.

The next major symptom of RLS is motor restlessness, often confused with akathisia. People who constantly move their legs while sitting or are fidgety do not necessarily have RLS. In RLS, the movements typically reduce or relieve the symptoms of RLS and these movements may vary from frequent tossing and turning of legs, to rubbing legs or pacing up and down. Patients with RLS therefore may find prolonged travel in a fixed position, such as long-distance flights, particularly troublesome.

Patients often volunteer the information as to the worsening or emergence of RLS symptoms during rest, or during quiet wakefulness, such as sitting watching television at night. The lack of sleep caused by RLS may make patients unduly sleepy during quiet wakefulness but, paradoxically, motor restlessness may kept them awake. In some patients mental distraction may avert symptoms of RLS (Table 5.4).

In general, the course of the syndrome is progressive with up to 60% reporting that their symptoms become increasingly severe. However, it usually follows a relapsing and remitting course with remissions of up to a month, or it can simply remain static[5]. Symptoms may appear during pregnancy or can be exacerbated by pregnancy (Table 5.5). The onset can occur

Table 5.4 Methods used by RLS patients to maintain relief from sensations/pain of RLS

Mental distraction
Hot or skin contact (compress, bath etc.) as counter stimulus
Massaging of legs/foot
Short naps throughout the day

Table 5.5 Pregnancy-related RLS

Typically third trimester
May disappear after delivery
May unmask chronic RLS
Often related to low iron or low folate

at any age, although the prevalence tends to increase with age; 42% of cases present before the age of 20. If asked about at presentation, many patients with idiopathic RLS report certain symptoms that date back to childhood and historically there is an association with 'growing pains' or hyperactivity as children.

Another distinguishing factor is that RLS is generally not associated with any abnormalities on neurologic examination. However, there is a relationship between RLS and neuropathy, mostly in those who have an older age of onset (Table 5.6).

Some patients with chronic, poorly-treated RLS may have symptoms during both day and night and the circadian pattern is lost. Unless the physician has a high index of suspicion, such patients are often thought to have neuropsychiatric problems rather than RLS[9,10].

Restless hands syndrome (RHS) mimics symptoms of RLS in the upper limb, typically the fingers, palm and wrist. Motor restlessness may be more evident on examination/inspection. Isolated RHS is rare and usually RHS develops as RLS becomes chronic or augmentation develops (see later)[10].

There are a few important further associations with RLS, which may aid the clinical diagnosis (Table 5.7). A higher body mass index, lower income, smoking, lack of exercise, low alcohol intake and diabetes mellitus have been identified as associated features in large study groups in both the US

Table 5.6 Neuropathy in contrast to RLS

Older age associated with axonal injury
Chronic, often painful
Usually non-familial
Usually normal ferritin level

Table 5.7 Observational and epidemiological studies suggest RLS may be associated with

High body mass index
Low income status
Smoking
Low alcohol consumption
Diabetes mellitus

and Europe. There is a slight predilection for women, and different racial groups may have varying frequencies of occurrence of RLS. There may also be associations with both neuropyschiatric problems and somatic complaints such as heart failure and hypertension[11].

Key points for the diagnosis of RLS include:

- The sensory symptoms of RLS
- Worse at night or at rest
- Improves with movement

There are some practical functional consequences of severe RLS, which clinicians may identify. These include:

- Daytime sleepiness
- Feeling tired
- Feeling depressed
- Poor concentration
- Fear of travel (long-distance airline travel).

DIFFERENTIAL DIAGNOSIS OF RLS

The secondary causes of RLS are discussed in another chapter. However, it is important to bear in mind that there are a few conditions that may masquerade as RLS. Therefore, in addition to a good history, investigations may be required to rule out other causes. Table 5.8 highlights the differential diagnoses of RLS[1,3,5].

Table 5.8   The most common differential diagnoses of RLS

General disorders
    Nocturnal leg cramps
    Akathisia
    Burning feet syndrome/small fiber neuropathy
    Dystonia in feet or toes
    Painful legs and moving toes
    Panic attacks
    Vascular disease (varicose veins, DVT, intermittent claudication)
    Vesper's curse

Sleep-related disorders
    Insomnia
    REM sleep behavior disorder
    Sleep apnea syndrome
    Sleep onset myoclonus

Nocturnal leg cramps may be described in a similar manner to RLS but important distinguishing features may be that there is no relationship with rest or relief on activity. In a UK survey, it was reported that many RLS patients are erroneously diagnosed as suffering from leg cramps and thereby prescribed inappropriate medications.

An uncommon condition, called painful legs and moving toes, causes pain in the legs in a very similar distribution to that of RLS, with, as the name suggests, involuntary movement of the toes but the pain is not relieved by movement. Nocturnal leg pain can be initiated by congestive heart failure in a condition called 'Vesper's curse' caused by engorgement of lumbar veins at night leading to transient stenosis of the lumbar cord, when the pain may extend to the lumbosacral region[5].

Akathisia is another important differential diagnosis. At times akathisia is very difficult to distinguish from RLS particularly as it may occur in PD. Akathisia may present as generalized involuntary movements without any sensory complaints and occurs at any time of day; it is associated with neuroleptic use, which may independently be a cause of secondary RLS (Table 5.9).

Another important differential diagnosis is that of polyneuropathy. The distinction between this and RLS lies with clinical examination and neurophysiologic tests (nerve conduction studies). However, a very important point to bear in mind is that it is possible for both RLS and polyneuropathy to occur concomitantly. The presence of PLMS or PLMW tends to suggest RLS. An indication that both disorders are present is that the sensory symptoms of polyneuropathy alone do not improve when the patient moves.

Table 5.9 The differences between akathisia and RLS

	Akathisia	RLS
Motor restlessness	All the time	At rest/sleep
Circadian rhythm	Nil	Present
Etiology	Neuroleptics Dopaminergic dysfunction	Dopaminergic drugs used to treat PD
Site	Face/tongue/upper limb Lower limbs	Usually lower limb
Movements	Fast and choleric	Slow and repetitive
Relief	Non-specific Occasionally movement	Movement

THE RELATIONSHIP BETWEEN RLS AND PARKINSON'S DISEASE

It has been suggested that up to 20% of Parkinson's disease (PD) patients also suffer from RLS[6,12]. It is difficult to decipher the relationship between the two disorders because there have not been many published studies looking closely at the relationship between them; RLS is treated by dopaminergic drugs used to treat PD, and RLS may be similar to other night-time problems occurring in PD, such as akathisia and nocturnal motor fluctuations.

The association between the two disorders may, however, add strength to the dopaminergic hypothesis of the causation of RLS. The areas especially implicated are the nigrostriatal system and the mesocorticolimbic systems, and interference with supraspinal dopaminergic inhibitory impulses leading to spinal flexor reflexes are also believed to be involved in the pathogenesis of RLS. Another aspect of the relationship between RLS and PD worthy of note is the fact that individuals with RLS who have been treated with levodopa develop augmentation and rebound. These phenomena are remarkably similar to the motor fluctuations which occur in PD treated long-term with levodopa.

The symptoms that PD sufferers complain of with regard to RLS-like symptoms are those of difficulty in sleeping – especially fragmented sleep and daytime somnolence which may be attributable to RLS itself – and/or motor, sensory and neuropyschiatric problems. PD patients also suffer from PLMS and it has been suggested that it occurs with increased frequency in PD, with an estimated 15% suffering from the disorder. Furthermore, central/?spinal cord related dopamine deficiency is thought to be the possible underlying cause of PLMS[13,14].

The clinician therefore needs to be aware of RLS occurring in PD as such symptoms may need individual treatment.

REFERENCES

1. Earley CJ. Clinical practice. Restless legs syndrome. *N Engl J Med* 2003; 348:2103–9

2. Tings T, Baier PC, Paulus W, *et al.* Restless legs syndrome induced by impairment of sensory spinal pathways. *J Neurol* 2003;250:499–500

3. Comella CL. Sleep disturbances in Parkinson's disease. *Curr Neurol Neurosci Rep* 2003;3:173–80

4. Appiah-Kubi L, Pal S, Chaudhuri KR. Restless legs syndrome, Parkinson's disease and sustained dopaminergic therapy for RLS. *Sleep Med* 2002;3(Suppl 1):S51–5

5. Chaudhuri KR, Appiah-Kubi L, Trenkwalder C. Restless legs syndrome; diagnosis and management. *J Neurol Neurosurg Psychiatry* 2001;71:143–6

6. Mandal S, Appiah-Kubi L, Porter MC, Chaudhuri KR. A clinical observational study of restless legs syndrome in Parkinson's disease. *Mov Disord* 2002;17(Suppl 5):S229

7. Ekbom, KA. Restless legs. *Acta Med Scand Suppl*, 1945;158:1–123

8. Montplaisir J, Boucher S, Poirier G, *et al.* Clinical polysomnographic and genetic characteristics of restless legs syndrome: a study of 133 patients diagnosed with new standard of criteria. *Mov Disord* 1997;1:61–5

9. Yoakum R. Night walkers: do your legs seem to have a life of their own? Your torment has a name. *Mod Maturity* 1994;55:82–4

10. Chaudhuri KR. Restless legs syndrome. Under-recognised and poorly treated. *Pract Neurol* 2003;3:204–13

11. Tan E-K, Ondo W. Restless legs syndrome: clinical features and treatment. *Am J Med Sci* 2000;319:397–403

12. Ondo WG, Vuong KD, Jankovic J. Exploring the relationship between Parkinson's disease and restless legs syndrome. *Arch Neurol* 2002;59:421–4

13. Rye DB, Jankovic J. Emerging views of dopamine in modulating sleep/wake state from an unlikely source: PD. *Neurology* 2002;58:341–6

14. Rye DB. Modulation of normal and pathologic motoneuron activity during sleep: insights from the neurology clinic, Parkinson's disease, and comments on parkinsonian-related sleepiness. *Sleep Med* 2002;3(Suppl):S43–9

6   *Secondary restless legs syndrome*

W. Ondo

In 1995, the International Restless Legs Syndrome Study Group described a set of minimal inclusion criteria for restless legs syndrome (RLS) consisting of four cardinal features: (1) desire to move the extremities, often associated with paresthesia/dysesthesia; (2) motor restlessness; (3) worsening of symptoms at rest and at least temporary relief with activity; and (4) worsening of symptoms in the evening or night[1]. Other features frequently associated with RLS include periodic limb movements while asleep (PLMS), a normal neurological examination, a tendency for symptoms to gradually worsen with age and improvement with dopaminergic treatments.

RLS is extremely common, effecting 5–10% of Caucasian populations, although it appears less common in Asian and African populations[2]. In roughly 60% of cases, a family history of RLS can be found, although this is often not initially reported by the patient[3]. Two gene loci have been published, although specific causative proteins remain elusive[4,5]. Given the wide distribution of RLS, however, it is likely that additional specific genetic etiologies are yet to be discovered. Despite the appropriate attention given to RLS genetics, between 2% and 6% of the population probably suffer from RLS without any identifiable highly penetrant genetic pattern. It is not known whether some 'genetic' forms of RLS could express low penetrance and mimic a sporadic pattern of onset. Currently, however, there is no evidence to support this pattern of penetrance[6]. Therefore, patients without a positive family history are classified as either primary RLS, if no other explanation is found, or secondary RLS, if they concurrently possess a condition known to be associated with RLS.

Correctly associating other medical conditions with a syndrome as common as RLS can be problematic, especially since RLS pathophysiology has been obscure. In fact, approximately 20 medical associations have been reported in the literature. Most of these are likely to be chance occurrences, owing to the past underestimated prevalence of RLS. Several medical conditions, however, are strongly associated with and possibly cause symptoms that are identical or nearly identical with those seen in 'genetic' or 'idiopathic' RLS. We will call these secondary RLS.

Since the exact pathophysiology of RLS is unknown, the relationship between 'idiopathic' RLS and 'secondary' RLS has not been elucidated in any case. It is not known why some persons with an associated medical condition develop RLS symptoms whereas others, usually most others, do not. Furthermore, it is not established whether persons with a genetic predisposition for RLS may be symptom-free without an additional deficit caused by an associated condition, or whether sub-clinical or mild genetic RLS is exacerbated by the coincidental occurrence of a secondary cause. Some speculate that multiple genes and multiple secondary medical conditions may contribute to the RLS phenotype in all patients; however, the exact interplay between genetics and environment is not known.

The most common causes of secondary RLS include renal failure, iron deficiency, neuropathy, myelinopathy, pregnancy and possibly Parkinson's disease. The majority of this chapter will concentrate on these. There is some evidence to support an association of RLS with tremor, some genetic ataxias, sleep apnea, fibromyalgia and rheumatological diseases. A variety of other associations are at best tenuous. Finally, several medications are known to exacerbate existing RLS or possibly to precipitate RLS themselves.

NEUROPATHY AND RLS

Numerous forms of neuropathy, including diabetic, alcoholic, amyloid, motor neuron disease, poliomyelitis and radiculopathy, have been associated with RLS[3,7–17]. Investigating the association of RLS and neuropathy, however, is very problematic. The definition of neuropathy varies in different studies. Some include only neuropathy diagnosed by standard electrophysiologic methods, which detect large fiber neuropathy. Others use a variety of physiologic studies with less established normative data, or even biopsies to capture abnormalities in small fiber nerves. These identify more patients with neuropathy; however, the prevalence of neuropathy in a general population without RLS is also very high using these criteria. Referral bias may also affect results since neuropathy patients with positive symptoms (RLS or pain) are more likely to seek medical attention than those with pure sensory loss. Finally, these are two very common conditions and a high number of patients with both would be expected randomly.

Several series have looked at RLS in populations of patients presenting with neuropathy. One retrospective study that evaluated 800 diabetic patients for neuropathic features reported that only 8.8% complained of RLS[13]. This was not significantly greater than 7% of controls. Interestingly, the percentage of type II diabetics affected by RLS was significantly more than type I diabetics ($p = 0.02$). This difference, however, may have resulted from the older age of the type II population. A prospective study evaluating consecutive patients with electrophysiologically diagnosed neuropathy reported that 8/154 (5%) met IRLSSG clinical criteria for RLS[14]. Symptoms improved with L-dopa in five patients. Interestingly, the RLS symptoms in two patients with Lyme-disease-associated neuropathy improved after antibiotic treatment. Although the authors felt that this represented an association of neuropathy and RLS, the 5% prevalence is actually lower than that usually reported in the general population.

Specific forms of neuropathy may incur different risks for the development of RLS. Gemignani and colleagues reported that 10/27 (37%) of patient with Charcot–Marie–Tooth type II (CMT II), an axonal neuropathy, had RLS, whereas RLS was not seen in any of 17 patients with CMT I, a demyelinating neuropathy[7]. The presence of RLS in CMT II correlated with other positive sensory symptoms such as pain. The same group has also suggested that symmetrical sensory neuropathies and female gender may predict RLS, at least in essential mixed cryoglobulinemia[8].

In contrast, studies that evaluated for neuropathy in populations of patients presenting with RLS suggest a more robust association. Iannoccone and co-workers initially suggested that all cases of RLS might have resulted from peripheral neuropathy too subtle to detect by standard electrophysiologic testing[10]. They reported at least one neuropathic abnormality in each of eight 'idiopathic' RLS patients, employing a battery of electrophysiologic and thermal sensitivity tests and sural nerve biopsies. This study, however, suffered from small sample size and poorly-defined normal parameters. Subsequent evaluation did yield some patients in whom no evidence of neuropathy could be demonstrated.

In our series, 37/98 (36.6%) of RLS patients demonstrated electrophysiologic evidence of neuropathy using standard EMG/NCV techniques. Most of these had mild-to-moderate sensory axonal neuropathies; however, the exact etiologies varied. Many of these patients demonstrated no evidence of neuropathy on clinical examination. The presence of neuropathy was much higher in patients who did not have a family history of RLS, compared with those who did have a family history: 22/31 (71%) vs.15/67 (24%), $p < 0.001$. Another four of those nine non-familial RLS with normal EMG examinations had very low ferritin levels, possibly accounting for their RLS. This suggests, but does not prove, that neuropathy does cause a true secondary form of RLS.

Small fiber neuropathy, which is only detectable on biopsy, is also found in a large number of patients presenting with RLS. Polydefkis and associates evaluated 22 RLS patients without risk factors for neuropathy using EMG/NVC and skin biopsies[11]. Of these, three had a purely large fiber neuropathy, three had a purely small fiber neuropathy, and two had mixed neuropathies. As in our results, RLS patients with neuropathy usually did not have a positive family history. Their RLS symptoms also began at an older age. Small fiber neuropathy can be difficult to accurately determine and requires biopsy and special stains to definitively diagnose (Figure 6.1). Currently, there is no compelling evidence to support this evaluation in the routine management of RLS.

The phenotype of neuropathic RLS may be slightly different from that of idiopathic RLS[3,11]. In our population, neuropathic RLS symptoms initially presented more acutely and at an older age, and then progressed much more rapidly. A large number of patients with neuropathic RLS reached maximum symptom intensity within 1 year from the initial symptom onset, which is unusual in idiopathic cases. Idiopathic RLS tended to begin with sensations in between the ankle and knee, whereas neuropathic RLS tended to initially occur distally or randomly throughout the leg. Neuropathic RLS may also have accompanying neuropathic pain, which is often burning and more superficial. The painful component and the urge to move, are seldom differentiated by the patient; they may, however, respond differently to treatment. The classic RLS urge to move and PLMS improve with dopaminergics, whereas the painful component usually requires other treatments, such as gabapentin or opioids. Finally, we have recently reported that neuropathic RLS patients are less likely to develop augmentation with chronic dopaminergic treatment[18] (Figure 6.2).

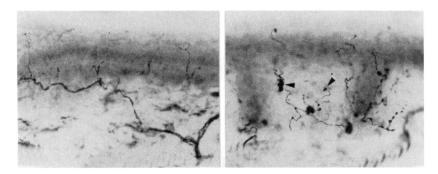

Figure 6.1 Small fiber neuropathy in restless legs syndrome. Left, normal thigh; right, neuropathy thigh

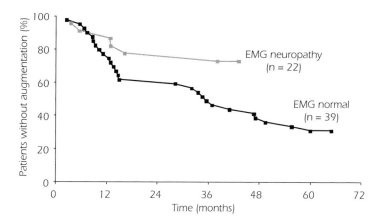

Figure 6.2 Survival curve for augmentation as a function of neuropathy status

Augmentation, as defined by any of: (1) an earlier onset of symptoms; (2) a greater symptom intensity; (3) an expanded anatomic involvement; or (4) reduced symptom relief with movement, represents the major problem with chronic dopaminergic therapies. Neuropathic RLS patients, however, might be more easily managed with dopaminergics over long periods of time.

Despite these phenotypic differences, it is impossible to clinically diagnosis neuropathic RLS accurately. We generally obtain an EMG/NCV in all cases of RLS, although their utility is debatable in cases with a strong family history and absent clinical signs of neuropathy on examination. If a neuropathy is discovered, a proper investigation of underlying and potentially treatable conditions is warranted.

The clinical similarities between neuropathic and idiopathic RLS suggest a common pathogenesis. Both animal models[19–21] and clinical movement disorders[22–24] suggest that permanent perturbation of CNS neurotransmitter function can follow a peripheral nervous system injury. Peripherally-induced RLS may similarly cause a CNS alteration since most evidence suggests CNS pathology in RLS. Alternatively, normal afferent stimulation, which is lacking in neuropathy, may mask latent RLS symptoms in all people. For example, patients with RLS will rub their legs or use hot water to increase afferent input in order to suppress symptoms. Better understanding of the exact relationship between RLS and neuropathy awaits more detailed epidemiology data and a better understanding of RLS pathogenesis as a whole.

MYELENOPATHY AND RLS

The spinal cord is strongly implicated in the pathogenesis of RLS[25,26]. This is based upon physiological data suggesting reduced inhibition at that level, anatomical theories and experimental models, and frequent cases of RLS and PLMS seen after transient or permanent spinal cord lesions. To date, no specific anatomy within the spinal cord is implicated in secondary RLS. Some feel that any deafferentation can result in RLS, whereas others have postulated that descending inhibitory tract dysfunction specifically causes RLS. Spinal cord blocks used for anesthesia are frequently reported to cause or exacerbate RLS[27,28]. Traumatic spinal cord lesions[29,30], neoplastic spinal lesions[31], demyelinating or post-infectious lesions[32–34] and syringomyelia[35] also precipitate RLS and PLMS.

Högl and colleagues systematically evaluated RLS following spinal anesthesia[27]. Of 161 subjects without any history of RLS, 8.7% developed RLS immediately after the procedure. Symptoms lasted for an average of 33 ± 30 days and were associated with low mean corpuscular volume and mean corpuscular hemoglobin. They felt that deafferentation might cause RLS in patients who were somehow predisposed.

One study specifically reported that demyelinating RLS responded well to dopaminergics[36]. Another study suggested that increased activity improved RLS and PLMS in subjects with complete cord injuries[29]. Large treatment studies, however, for either RLS of PLMS in this population are lacking.

UREMIA AND RLS

Uremia secondary to renal failure is strongly associated with RLS symptoms. Several series report a 20–57% prevalence of RLS in renal dialysis patients; however, only a minority of uremic patients volunteer RLS symptoms unless specifically queried[37–56] (Table 6.1). The prevalence of RLS in mild to moderate renal failure that does not require dialysis is unknown.

The pathogenesis of uremic RLS is unclear, as different series have reported a variety of specific associations. The importance of the degree of renal failure, as measured by creatine clearance, is also not clear. One study reported that RLS was associated with higher blood urea nitrogen (BUN) and creatine[57], but another actually reported that insomnia and RLS were associated with a lower BUN and creatine[48]. The majority of series, however, have not found any association with either marker of renal function. One retrospective study in 'normal' elderly patients without renal failure

Table 6.1   Studies evaluating restless legs syndrome in renal failure

Author	Cohort	RLS diagnosis	# and % with RLS	RLS predictors
Takaki et al.[*] (2003)[60]	HD	IRLSSG (4/4)	60/490 (12.2%)	Hyperphosphatemia Stress
		IRLSSG (≥ 2/4)	112//490 (22.9%)	
Cirignotta et al. (2002)[62]	HD	Written questionnaire IRLSSG interview	/127 (50%) /127 (33.3%)	NR
Sabbatini et al. (2002)[48]	HD	RLS question	257/694 (37%)	None
Hui et al. (2000)[42]	PD	Written question	124/201 (62%)	Insomnia
Virga et al. (1998)[51]	HD	'RLS'	(27.4%)	None
Collado-Seidel et al. (1998)[39]	HD	IRLSSG (4/4)	32/138 (23%)	Inc. parathyroid hormone
		IRLSSG (≥ 3/4)	44/138 (32%)	
Winkelmann et al. (1995)[53]	HD	IRLSSG (3/4)	/204 (20%)	None Dec. Hct Poor sleep
Walker et al. (1995)[50]	HD	ICSD	31/54 (57%)	Inc. BUN, $p = 0.04$ Inc. Cr, $p = 0.08$
Stepanski et al. (1995)[49]	PD	'Leg twitching'	26/81 (32%)	NR
Holley et al. (1992)[41]	HD PD	'RLS'	30/70 (42%)	NR
Roger et al. (1991)[47]	HD PD	'RLS'	22/55 (40%)	Hct, $p = 0.03$ Female
Bastani (1987)[146]	HD	'RLS'	6/42 (17%)	NR
Nielsen (1971)[86]	None	'RLS'	43/109 (39%)	NR

correlated PLMS with high normal BUN[58], but a subsequent prospective study by the same group found no correlation between PLMS and creatinine clearance[59].

Roger and co-workers correlated RLS in dialysis patients with a lower hematocrit, and in their population the RLS improved after the administration of erythropoietin[47]. Neither iron studies nor renal function correlated with symptoms. In fact, no study has clearly implicated an association of low iron stores and RLS within a uremic RLS population. It should be noted, however, that iron regulation is markedly abnormal in dialysis patients. It can be difficult to determine because ferritin levels are often artificially elevated as an acute phase reactant, and most dialysis patients now receive erythropoietin, which can affect iron metabolism. Therefore, it is difficult to accurately assess whether iron abnormalities may underlie RLS in the dialysis population.

The most extensive study of RLS in dialysis patients reported that 23% of 126 dialysis patients had definite RLS whereas 32% had probable RLS[39]. The authors attempted to correlate the presence of RLS with numerous factors including age, duration of uremia and need for dialysis, time on dialysis per week, hemoglobin, hematocrit, erythrocytes, s-ferritin, s-transferrin, s-iron, calcium, standard biochemical indices and parathyroid hormone (iPTH) levels. They did not assess neuropathy. Interestingly, the only feature that correlated with RLS was significantly lower iPTH levels ($p < 0.01$). There was no association with calcium levels. The authors admit that they did not correct for multiple comparisons, and this data has not been replicated.

RLS in uremic patients is clearly associated with insomnia and neuropsychiatric sequelae. Takaki and colleagues evaluated 490 uremic patients on hemodialysis therapy in Japan for both social-psychiatric issues and physiologic measures[60]. They reported that 'hyperphosphatemia, anxiety, and a greater degree of "emotion-oriented coping with stress" were independently related to the presence of RLS, and concluded that the pathophysiology of RLS in this population is likely to be multi-factorial.

Both RLS and PLMS have been associated with increased mortality in the dialysis population[53,61]. In the most detailed study to evaluate this association, RLS was strongly associated with sleep abnormalities[53]. Both RLS and sleep abnormalities, along with transferrin saturation, predicted premature discontinuation from dialysis. It is unclear whether the high mortality in the RLS/dialysis population results from discontinuation of dialysis, or whether RLS is a biological marker of some factor that also predicts mortality.

Dialysis patients suffer from numerous sleep problems and RLS can be easily confused with other sensory-motor phenomena experienced by dialysis patients such as pruritus. It is therefore difficult to diagnose RLS in this population without personal interrogation[62]. Nevertheless, the RLS seen in dialysis patients is often severe. Wetter and co-workers compared clinical and polysomnographic features of idiopathic RLS and uremic RLS in a large clinical series[52]. They reported no differences in sensory symptoms but noted increased dyskinesia while awake (78% vs. 51%) and statistically significant greater numbers of PLMS in uremic RLS patients. Uremic RLS patients subjectively rated their sleep as worse than idiopathic RLS patients; however, sleep architecture and duration were similar on polysomnograms. They found no differences in treatment responses, as both groups responded best to L-dopa.

There is no study directly comparing RLS experienced with hemodialysis and RLS seen in peritoneal dialysis. Hui and associates, however, using a similar questionnaire on both groups, but reporting them separately, diagnosed RLS in 70% of 43 peritoneal dialysis patients[42] and 62% of 201 patients on hemodialysis[43]. There are potential differences in the underlying disease processes between these two groups, so a direct 'treatment' comparison is problematic.

Overall, dialysis does not improve RLS. In fact one study suggested that RLS correlated with greater dialysis frequency[44]. Patients who receive kidney transplants, however, usually experience dramatic improvement in RLS within days to weeks[63,64]. The degree of symptom alleviation appears to correlate with improved kidney function. Winkelmann and colleagues reported that all patients with successful transplantations ($n = 8$) initially had complete resolution of RLS symptoms within 3 weeks; however, symptoms gradually returned in three of these subjects over several years[64]. Patients in whom the transplant failed did not improve, and one patient who did not improve after a failed transplant did subsequently improve after a successful one. These observations suggest that the symptoms are directly related to the kidney failure rather than to immunosuppressive drugs, subclinical uremic neuropathy or other secondary phenomena.

Uremic RLS, when severe, is more refractory to pharmacologic treatment than idiopathic RLS. Dopaminergics are effective against uremic RLS[65]; however, relatively higher doses may be required. In fact, the only dopaminergic RLS treatment trial to not report robust positive results was low-dose pergolide (0.25 mg/night) in uremic RLS[46]. In the author's personal experience, if dopaminergics are ineffective, many uremic patients benefit from low-dose methadone. Gabapentin may also be helpful. Transplantation, when possible, may permanently alleviate RLS symptoms.

IRON DEFICIENCY AND RLS

Recent evidence strongly implicates brain iron abnormalities in all cases of RLS. CSF ferritin is lower in RLS cases[66], and imaging studies show reduced iron stores in the striatum and red nucleus[67] (Figure 6.3). Pathological data in RLS show reduced ferritin, iron staining and increased transferrin stains, but also reduced transferrin receptors[68]. This is important, because globally reduced iron stores would normally upregulate transferrin receptors. Therefore it appears that primary RLS has reduced intracellular iron indices secondary to a perturbation of homeostatic mechanisms that regulate iron influx and/or efflux from the cell. Several proposed mechanisms for this dysregulation are discussed elsewhere. Nevertheless, if low CNS intracellular iron causes RLS symptoms, it is intuitive to suggest that reduced body stores of iron could also result in low CNS intracellular iron and also cause RLS symptoms.

The mechanisms by which this low intracellular iron subsequently manifests RLS symptomatology are not well understood. Dopaminergic systems are strongly implicated in RLS. Most researchers agree that dopamine agonists most robustly treat RLS symptoms and dopaminergic functional brain imaging studies inconsistently show modest abnormalities[69–71]. There are several interactions between iron and dopamine. First, iron is a co-factor for tyrosine-hydroxylase, which is the rate-limiting step in the production of dopamine. Iron chelation reduces dopamine transporter (DAT) protein

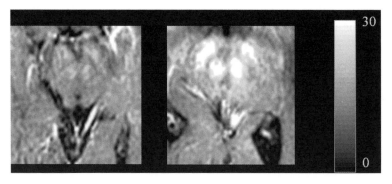

Figure 6.3 MRI sequenced to show iron as bright areas in normal control (left) and patient with RLS (right)

expression and activity in mice[72]. Second, iron is a component of the dopamine type-2 (D2) receptor. Iron deprivation in rats results in a 40–60% reduction of D2 post-synaptic receptors[73,74]. The effect is quite specific, as other neurotransmitter systems including D1 receptors are not affected. Third, iron is involved in Thy1 protein regulation. This cell adhesion molecule, which is robustly expressed on dopaminergic neurons, is reduced in brain homogenates in iron-deprived mice[75]. Thy1 regulates vesicular release of monoamines, including dopamine[76]. It also stabilizes synapses and suppresses dendritic growth[77]. At the behavioral level, iron deficiency blocks apomorphine, a dopamine agonist, inducing behavioral responses in rats[78,79].

A possible association between RLS symptoms and systemic iron deficiency has long been recognized[80–84]. Ekbom originally reported that about 25% of his RLS patients were iron deficient[83]. One study that evaluated a population of 80 iron-deficient patients reported that 43% of them complained of symptoms of RLS[82]. In fact, treatment of RLS with intravenous iron was successfully employed 50 years ago. Unfortunately, the importance of this groundbreaking research was only realized in the past decade when this association was rediscovered.

A series of recent reports have associated low serum ferritin levels with RLS[66,67,85–89]. Low serum ferritin levels are the best indicator of low iron stores, although high ferritin levels do not necessarily indicate adequate iron stores, since ferritin is an acute-phase reactant. Therefore, in some inflammatory settings, such as renal failure, low iron stores can be difficult to identify. Each ferritin molecule can hold 2000–3000 iron atoms. Serum-free elemental iron levels fluctuate markedly throughout the day and are therefore not a useful measure. Transferrin helps identify excessive iron but does not accurately identify reduced iron stores. Therefore, when screening for low systemic iron stores in RLS, ferritin is the most meaningful test.

In the modern era, O'Keeffe and associates were the first to report on ferritin levels in 18 elderly patients with symptomatic RLS and compared them with age-matched controls[86]. They discovered significantly lower ferritin levels in affected patients. Serum iron, hemoglobin levels, B_{12} and folate did not differ between the groups. Serum ferritin levels and symptom severity (determined by a simple ten-point subjective scale) were also inversely correlated (Spearman's ρ –0.53, $p < 0.05$). Two months of oral iron supplementation improved the subjective scores in most affected patients. The authors suggested that all RLS patients with ferritin levels below 50 ng/ml (a level within the normal range) should receive iron supplementation.

Sun and co-workers[87] reported that RLS severity and awakening from PLMS were greater in RLS patients with lower serum ferritin levels (< or = 50 ng/ml) compared with those with higher serum ferritins (total n = 27). Silber and co-workers[88]. reported on eight patients whose RLS started shortly after donating blood. All had low serum ferritins and some were anemic. They suggested that RLS might be a relative contraindication against donating blood.

In contrast, the MEMO study was a population-based survey of 365 German subjects, aged 65–83. Serum ferritin, as evaluated by quartile analysis, was not significantly different in the 9.8% who met criteria for RLS, compared with the remaining population[90]. Although these data represent a superior design to study this question, a possible association may have been missed because of the relatively low number of RLS cases.

Low serum iron may only be associated with certain populations of RLS patients. We have reported that serum ferritin is lower in patients with RLS who lack a family history compared with those with familial RLS[85,91]. Serum ferritin in RLS patients with a positive family history was 96.4 ± 64.5 ng/ml (n = 64) compared with 61.5 ± 54.1 ng/ml (n = 26) in patients without a family history of RLS.

Earley and colleagues have made the same general observation, but segregated the groups according to age of RLS onset[92]. The patients with an older age of RLS onset had lower serum ferritin levels compared with patients with a younger age of onset. These groups, however, generally represent the same dichotomy as genetic-based segregations, since there is a very strong correlation between age of onset of RLS and the presence of a family history of RLS. An older age at onset and non-familial RLS appear to be strongly associated with low serum ferritin levels, whereas a younger age at onset and familial RLS generally are not associated with low serum ferritin levels. Therefore the clinical epidemiology correlates nicely with the known basic science. Familial or primary RLS may be caused by CNS iron dysregulation; however, it can also be secondarily caused by systemic iron deficiency in people without a genetic cause for RLS.

Finally, it should be noted that two other secondary causes of RLS, pregnancy and renal failure, are also associated with iron deficiency. It is unclear whether this is in any way causal, since both of those scenarios improve with definitive treatments (delivery and renal transplant) more rapidly than serum iron deficits would be restored. Nevertheless, iron deficiency remains the most common denominator among the accepted secondary causes of RLS.

The role of iron replacement in iron-deficiency-associated RLS and in idiopathic RLS is under investigation. Although open-label oral iron supplementation has been reported to improve RLS[93], the only controlled study of oral iron supplementation failed to improve RLS symptoms[94]. Oral iron, however, has numerous limitations. It is very poorly absorbed and poorly tolerated. Absorption can be improved when the iron is taken within a moderately acidic milieu, which is practically achieved by the concurrent addition of ascorbic acid. Even with ideal compliance, only modest augmentations of serum ferritin levels are usually achieved with oral supplementation. In contrast, the administration of intravenous iron can dramatically increase serum ferritin levels. Nordlander first reported the benefit of intravenous iron[80]. More recently an open-label study has also demonstrated robust efficacy[95]. Additional studies are ongoing.

PREGNANCY

The development of RLS during pregnancy has long been recognized. Ekbom originally reported that 11% of 500 pregnant women had RLS[84]. In pregnant women who were iron deficient, as measured by a serum iron level of < 600 μg/l, this rose to 24%. Goodman and co-workers reported that 19% of 500 women at 32–34 weeks' gestation suffered from RLS[96]. Symptoms were mild in most cases. Only 16 of the 97 affected women reported RLS prior to pregnancy, and all but 6 of the 97 reported complete cessation of RLS symptoms by 10 days postpartum.

Manconi and associates recently evaluated risk factors for RLS in 606 pregnancies[97]. They reported that 26% of these women suffered with RLS, usually in the last trimester. In contrast to the Goodman cohort, 42% of affected women experienced RLS symptoms at some point prior to their pregnancy. The authors could find no significant differences in age, pregnancy duration, mode of delivery, tobacco use, the woman's body mass index, baby weight or iron/folate supplementation in those with RLS. Hemoglobin, however, was significantly lower in the RLS group, and plasmatic iron tended to be lower, compared with those without RLS.

Lee and colleagues reported that 23% of 29 third-trimester women developed RLS during pregnancy[98]. The RLS resolved shortly postpartum in all but one subject. Women with RLS in their population demonstrated lower preconception levels of ferritin but were similar to women without RLS during pregnancy. In contrast, the subjects with RLS maintained lower serum folate levels throughout pregnancy. Botez also reported an association of RLS and lower serum folate levels[99].

The relationship between RLS during pregnancy and RLS later in life is not clear. Winkelman and co-workers found that 19.1% of women with hereditary RLS reported an exacerbation of RLS during pregnancy compared with only 2.6% who had RLS, but lacked a family history of it[100]. This might be attributable to the younger age of onset in the hereditary RLS. Finally, multiple pregnancies may be a risk factor for the development of late-life RLS in all subjects (Winkelmann, personal communication).

Pharmacological treatment of RLS during pregnancy can be problematic. Benzodiazepines are relatively contraindicated. Dopaminergics have not been clearly associated with birth defects; however, there is little experience with their use and they are rated as category C during pregnancy. Low doses of some opioids are probably the safest treatment in this population. High doses can result in neonatal withdrawal syndromes.

PARKINSON'S DISEASE AND RLS

RLS and Parkinson's disease (PD) both respond to dopaminergic treatments, both show dopaminergic abnormalities on functional imaging[71,101] and both are associated with PLMS[102]. We now know that the pathology of the two dopaminergically-treated diseases are very different and, in regard to iron accumulation, actually quite opposite[68]. Nevertheless, a relationship between the two conditions has long been sought. Results, however, have been mixed. Prior to the development of IRLSSG criteria, some studies[103,104], but not others[105,106], have found a higher prevalence of RLS in patients with PD.

In a survey of 303 consecutive PD patients, we found that 20.8% of all patients with PD met the diagnostic criteria for RLS[85]. Very similar findings have recently been reported by other groups (Chaudhuri, personal communication). Despite this high number of cases, there are several caveats that tend to lessen its clinical significance. The RLS symptoms in PD patients are often ephemeral, usually not severe, and can be confused with other PD symptoms such as wearing-off dystonia, akathisia or internal tremor. Furthermore, most patients in our group were not previously diagnosed with RLS and few recognized that this was separate from other PD symptoms.

After determining the prevalence of RLS in PD, we next evaluated for factors that could predict RLS in this population, and determined that only lower serum ferritin levels predicted RLS symptoms in the PD population (Table 6.2). RLS did not correlate with duration of PD, age, Hoehn and Yahr staging of PD, gender, dementia, use of levodopa, use of dopamine agonists, history of pallidotomy or history of deep brain stimulation (DBS). PD symptoms preceded RLS symptoms in 35/41 (85.4%, $\chi^2(1) = 20.5$, $p < 0.0001$) of cases in which patients confidently remembered the initial onset of both symptoms. Only 22/109 (20.2%) of all RLS/PD patients reported a positive family history of RLS, compared with more than 60% of our non-PD RLS population. The serum ferritin was also lower in the PD/RLS group compared with the idiopathic RLS group. In these cases with PD who did have a family history of RLS, the RLS symptoms usually preceded PD and generally resembled typical RLS. In short, our results do not suggest that RLS is a *forme fruste* or a risk factor for the subsequent development of PD, but rather that PD is a risk factor for RLS, which might constitute an under-recognized non-motor feature of PD.

Krishnan and associates evaluated the prevalence of RLS in patients with PD compared with normal controls in a population from India[107]. Interestingly, they found that found that 10 of 126 cases of PD (7.9%) vs. only 1 of 128 controls (0.8%, $p = 0.01$) reported RLS. PD patients with RLS were older and reported more depression. Although both prevalences are lower than US reports, the difference in RLS prevalence between PD and controls is similar. This probably reflects baseline epidemiology that suggests RLS is less common in non-Caucasian populations. Likewise Tan, in a mostly Chinese population in Singapore, found only a single case of RLS out of 125 patients presenting with PD[108]. He also reported a very low RLS prevalence in the general population[2].

Evaluating the prevalence of PD in populations presenting with RLS is problematic, since PD symptoms would usually be more overt and precipitate an evaluation. Banno and co-workers, however reported that 20% of RLS patients had 'extrapyramidal signs'[104]. Fazzini and colleagues reported that 19/29 RLS patients had PD symptoms[109]. In the author's experience, RLS does not predispose to the development of PD; however, definitive prospective epidemiology does not exist for this scenario.

TREMOR

In our movement disorder clinic, we frequently see postural tremor in patients referred for RLS. Two major categories have been observed. RLS patients without any family history of tremor often have mild postural

Table 6.2 Data regarding RLS in PD

	Original PD without RLS (n = 240)	Original PD/ RLS cohort (n = 63)	Total PD/ RLS group (n = 109)	Total 'RLS only' group (n = 146)	'RLS only' (+) Family history of RLS (n = 96)	'RLS only' (−) Family history of RLS (n = 50)
Age (years)	67.5 ± 11.0	67.0 ± 9.8	67.9 ± 10.0	59.8 ± 15.1	59.3 ± 14.9	60.9 ± 15.6
Age onset of RLS (years)	N/A	62.5 ± 12.8	56.6 ± 18.6	35.6 ± 19.8‡	29.8 ± 17.5	46.5 ± 19.5
Percentage with a (+) family history of RLS	—	17.5	20.2	65.8**	100	0
Percentage male	62.5	52.4	48.6	37.0	35.4	40.0
Ferritin (ng/ml)	88.4 ± 67.5* (n = 32)	50.7 ± 46.6 (n = 25)	58.8 ± 51.0 (n = 46)	86.3 ± 63.0† (n = 90)	96.4 ± 64.5 (n = 64)	61.5 ± 54.1 (n = 26)

*$p < 0.05$, $t$test, PD without RLS vs. PD with RLS; †$p < 0.01$, ANOVA, PD with RLS vs. RLS only; ‡$p < 0.0001$, χ^2PD with RLS vs. RLS only; **$p < 0.0001$, ANOVA, PD with RLS vs. RLS only

tremor on examination. Usually they do not suffer any functional disability from this, and may not even appreciate the tremor until it is discussed. Physiologic studies to differentiate essential tremor from enhanced physiologic tremor have not been performed in this population. A second group of RLS patients have a family history of essential tremor. In fact, the family on which the 2p chromosome ET gene locus was identified had over 30 members who also complained of RLS[110]. There was a high, but not perfect, co-segregation between RLS and ET in this and other families. Anecdotally, we have implanted thalamic (VIM) deep-brain stimulators (DBS) into several ET/RLS patients to treat their tremor. Despite fair-to-excellent tremor control, VIM DBS does not seem to affect RLS symptoms. An association between RLS and ET has also been observed by some researchers[111], but not by others (Walters, personal communication).

ATAXIA

Abele and associates reported that RLS was seen in 28% of 58 subjects with genetic ataxias (SCA1, SCA-2, SCA-3)[112]. This was greater than the 10% reported by their control population. The average age at onset of RLS was 49 years. RLS did not correlate with the presence of neuropathy, or with CAG expansion length, but did correlate with the duration of neurological symptoms normally associated with those conditions.

Schols and co-workers reported that RLS was seen in 45% of patients with SCA-3 (Machado–Joseph disease), but was uncommon in other genetic ataxias[113]. They felt that RLS tended to be more common in patients with neuropathy, but it could also be seen without neuropathy. Family members without SCA-3 did not have any RLS symptoms. A separate report described RLS symptoms in a family with intermediate length CAG repeats for SCA-3[114]. There are no systematic reports of treatment for RLS in these populations.

RHEUMATOLOGIC CONDITIONS

RLS has been associated with rheumatoid arthritis (RA) in two separate series prior to the adoption of IRLSSG criteria[115,116]. Reynolds reported RLS symptoms in 30% of 70 patients with RA versus only 6% of 70 age-matched controls[115]. Salih and colleagues reported that 25% of 46 patients with RA met their RLS criteria versus 4% of 30 osteoarthritis controls[116]. Interestingly, RLS patients appeared to have had significantly lower ferritin levels than controls, and a mildly higher rate of neuropathy. These, however, were not commented upon by the authors. Another study, comparing sleep disturbances between patients with RA and Sjögren's syndrome, found that only 2% of 42 RA patients complained of 'restless legs' whereas, 24% of 40 Sjögren's patients reported this symptom ($p < 0.01$)[117]. These conflicting results may attest to difficulties in diagnosis within this population.

In contrast, we evaluated for rheumatologic serology abnormalities in 68 subjects presenting to a neurology/movement disorders clinic with RLS[91]. We did not find that either rheumatoid factor (RF) or SSA (Ro) / SSB (La) antibodies occurred more frequently than in the general population. A positive RF was seen in 3.6% of RLS patients and a positive SSA/SSB was seen in 3.1%. None of these subjects had overt evidence of rheumatologic disease; however, it should be noted that they were not examined by a rheumatologist. It is still therefore possible that subjects presenting with rheumatologic diseases could manifest RLS symptoms, but it should be pointed out that neither of the association studies employed current RLS criteria. Furthermore, pain from rheumatologic disease is often worse at night, and can improve with movement. The quality and location (joints) is different from RLS, but this is difficult to incorporate into formal disease inclusion criteria.

Fibromyalgia has also been associated with RLS[118,119]. In the author's opinion, it is difficult to make a separate diagnosis of RLS in patients with chronic pain conditions that often worsen at night, and cause insomnia. Further investigation of this association is warranted.

MISCELLANEOUS

Sleep apnea has been strongly associated with PLMS[120], but it is less clear that it is associated with RLS. Some feel that there is a strong association [Kushida, personal communication]; however, there is relatively little published literature to support this[121].

Numerous other conditions have been anecdotally associated with RLS. Some of these include Huntington's disease[122], hypothyroidism[123], chronic respiratory insufficiency[124], acute intermittent porphyria[125], partial gastrectomy[126], venous insufficiency[127], varicose veins[128], peripheral microembolism[129], Tourette's syndrome[130], Isaac's syndrome[131], hypothyroidism[132] and telangiectasia[133]. In no case is there compelling evidence to suggest that these represent more than coincidental co-occurrence.

MEDICATION-EXACERBATED RLS

A variety of medications are implicated in exacerbating pre-existent RLS or directly causing RLS symptoms. This distinction can be difficult to determine, since latent RLS may first be noticed following ingestion of a precipitating medication. In no case is the exact etiology of medication-induced RLS known, but as a general rule medications that relax or sedate can worsen RLS.

Dopamine antagonists clearly worsen RLS in many cases[134–137]. This can be expected when one considers the robust efficacy of dopamine agonists used to treat RLS. Most clinicians are aware that anti-psychotics block dopamine; however, anti-nausea medications such as prochlorperazine (Compazine), metoclopramide (Reglan), promazine (Sparine), droperidol (Inapsine), promethazine (Phenergan) and trimethobenzamide (Tigan) also have strong antagonistic effects. We have seen marked exacerbation of RLS in hospitalized patients who are relatively immobile, especially in a leg cast, and receive anti-nausea or anti-pruritic dopamine antagonists. We once observed a patient who was misdiagnosed with delirium tremens and transferred to a psychiatry ward after receiving two doses of promethazine. After a single dose of levodopa she returned to normal.

Mirtazepine (Remeron) may particularly provoke RLS[138,139]. This unique anti-depressant is quite soporific. Among other mechanisms it is a potent 5-HT2a antagonist. Other 5-HT2a antagonists, including mianserin, are also reported to exacerbate RLS[140].

Serotonin re-uptake inhibitors have been found to exacerbate RLS[141,142], and improve RLS[143]. We do not feel that these medications are contraindicated in RLS, but do favor more stimulating anti-depressants. Lithium can worsen RLS[144,145] and in the author's opinion can worsen or even cause parkinsonism in addition to tremor.

Antihistamines, especially non-prescription drugs, may be the most common culpable agents. Persons often take these medications as sleeping aids only to find they stimulate their RLS symptoms. Individuals who are not cognizant of their RLS diagnosis may simply report that sleeping pills 'make them wired' or 'have an opposite effect'. Many anti-depressants used for sleep, such as amitriptyline, also have strong anti-histaminergic properties and can worsen RLS. Finally, even benzodiazepines, when not adequate to induce sleep, can actually worsen RLS sensory-motor phenomena. They still, however, may improve sleep efficiency.

CONCLUSION

Known secondary causes of RLS are abundant and account for a large number of RLS cases. In our evaluation of an RLS patient we always perform a detailed neurologic examination to look for other neurologic signs. We usually perform EMG/NCV to evaluate for neuropathy. If a neuropathy is found, then further evaluation including thyroid tests, B_{12}, folate, etc. is justified. We always test for serum ferritin levels and consider supplementation if they are relatively low. Estimation of basic electrolytes, to evaluate renal function, is also justified if not previously done. In certain clinical situations, we may perform additional rheumatologic evaluations. We have found little utility for imaging tests or further evaluation of possible secondary causes in patients clinically presenting with RLS.

REFERENCES

1.   Walters AS. Toward a better definition of the restless legs syndrome. The International Restless Legs Syndrome Study Group. *Mov Disord* 1995;10: 634–42

2.   Tan EK, Seah A, See SJ, *et al.* Restless legs syndrome in an Asian population: A study in Singapore. *Mov Disord* 2001;16:577–9

3.   Ondo W, Jankovic J. Restless legs syndrome: clinicoetiologic correlates. *Neurology* 1996;47:1435–41

4.   Bonati MT, Ferini-Strambi L, Aridon P, *et al.* Autosomal dominant restless legs syndrome maps on chromosome 14q. *Brain* 2003;126:1485–92

5.   Desautels A, Turecki G, Montplaisir J, *et al.* Evidence for a genetic association between monoamine oxidase A and restless legs syndrome. *Neurology* 2002;59:215–19

6.   Winkelmann J, Muller-Myhsok B, Wittchen HU, *et al.* Complex segregation analysis of restless legs syndrome provides evidence for an autosomal dominant mode of inheritance in early age at onset families. *Ann Neurol* 2002;52:297–302

7.   Gemignani F, Marbini A, Di Giovanni G, *et al.* Charcot-Marie-Tooth disease type 2 with restless legs syndrome. *Neurology* 1999;52:1064–6

8.   Gemignani F, Marbini A, Di Giovanni G, *et al.* Cryoglobulinaemic neuropathy manifesting with restless legs syndrome. *J Neurol Sci* 1997;152:218–23

9.   Frankel BL, Patten BM, Gillin JC. Restless legs syndrome. Sleep-electroencephalographic and neurologic findings. *JAMA* 1974;230:1302–3

10.   Iannaccone S, Zucconi M, Marchettini P, *et al.* Evidence of peripheral axonal neuropathy in primary restless legs syndrome. *Mov Disord* 1995;10:2–9

11. Polydefkis M, Allen RP, Hauer P, *et al.* Subclinical sensory neuropathy in late-onset restless legs syndrome. *Neurology* 2000;55:1115–21

12. Salvi F, Montagna P, Plasmati R, *et al.* Restless legs syndrome and nocturnal myoclonus: initial clinical manifestation of familial amyloid polyneuropathy. *J Neurol Neurosurg Psychiatry* 1990;53:522–5

13. O'Hare JA, Abuaisha F, Geoghegan M. Prevalence and forms of neuropathic morbidity in 800 diabetics. *Irish J Med Sci* 1994;163:132–5

14. Rutkove SB, Matheson JK, Logigian EL. Restless legs syndrome in patients with polyneuropathy. *Muscle Nerve* 1996;19:670–2

15. Harriman DG, Taverner D, Woolf AL. Ekbom's syndrome and burning paresthesiae: a biopsy study by vital staining and electron microscopy of the intramuscular innervation with a note on age changes in motor nerve endings. *Brain* 1970;93:393–406

16. Gorman CA, Dyck PJ, Pearson JS. Symptom of restless legs. *Arch Intern Med* 1965;115:155–60

17. Walters AS, Wagner M, Hening WA. Periodic limb movements as the initial manifestation of restless legs syndrome triggered by lumbosacral radiculopathy [Letter]. *Sleep* 1996;19:825–6

18. Ondo WG, Vuong K, Romanyshyn J. The long-term treatment of restless legs syndrome with dopamine agonists. *Neurology* 2003;60(Suppl 1):A290

19. Curtis R, Adryan KM, Zhu Y, *et al.* Retrograde axonal transport of ciliary neurotrophic factor is increased by peripheral nerve injury. *Nature* 1993; 365:253–5

20. Braune S, Schady W. Changes in sensation after nerve injury or amputation: the role of central factors. *J Neurol Neurosurg Psychiatry* 1993;56:393–9

21. Jenkins R, Hunt SP. Long-term increase in the levels of c-jun m RNA and Jun protein like immunoreactivity in motor and sensory neurons following axon damage. *Neurosci Lett* 1991;129:107–10

22. Ashizawa T, Cardoso F. Peripherally induced tremor and parkinsonism. *Mov Disord* 1995;10:103–5

23. Koller WC, Wong GF, Lang A. Posttraumatic movement disorders: a review. *Mov Disord* 1989;4:20–36

24. Jankovic J. Post-traumatic movement disorders: central and peripheral mechanisms [Comment]. *Neurology* 1994;44:2006–14

25. Ondo WG, He Y, Rajasekaran S, Le WD. Clinical correlates of 6-hydroxydopamine injections into A11 dopaminergic neurons in rats: a possible model for restless legs syndrome. *Mov Disord* 2000;15:154–8

26. Bara-Jimenez W, Aksu M, Graham B, *et al.* Periodic limb movements in sleep: state-dependent excitability of the spinal flexor reflex [Comment]. *Neurology* 2000;54:1609–16

27. Hogl B, Frauscher B, Seppi K, *et al.* Transient restless legs syndrome after spinal anesthesia: a prospective study. *Neurology* 2002;59:1705–7

28. Moorthy SS, Dierdorf SF. Restless legs during recovery from spinal anesthesia [Letter]. *Anesth Analg* 1990;70:337

29. de Mello MT, Lauro FA, Silva AC, Tufik S. Incidence of periodic leg movements and of the restless legs syndrome during sleep following acute physical activity in spinal cord injury subjects. *Spinal Cord* 1996;34:294–6

30. Hartmann M, Pfister R, Pfadenhauer K. Restless legs syndrome associated with spinal cord lesions [Letter]. *J Neurol Neurosurg Psychiatry* 1999;66:688–9

31. Lee MS, Choi YC, Lee SH, Lee SB. Sleep-related periodic leg movements associated with spinal cord lesions. *Mov Disord* 1996;11:719–22

32. Brown LK, Heffner JE, Obbens EA. Transverse myelitis associated with restless legs syndrome and periodic movements of sleep responsive to an oral dopaminergic agent but not to intrathecal baclofen. *Sleep* 2000;23:591–4

33. Bruno RL. Abnormal movements in sleep as a post-polio sequela. *Am J Phys Med Rehabil* 1998;77:339–43

34. Hemmer B, Riemann D, Glocker FX, *et al*. Restless legs syndrome after a borrelia-induced myelitis. *Mov Disord* 1995;10:521–2

35. Winkelmann J, Wetter TC, Trenkwalder C, Auer DP. Periodic limb movements in syringomyelia and syringobulbia. *Mov Disord* 2000;15:752–3

36. de Mello MT, Poyares DL, Tufik S. Treatment of periodic leg movements with a dopaminergic agonist in subjects with total spinal cord lesions. *Spinal Cord* 1999;37:634–7

37. Bhatia M, Bhowmik D. Restless legs syndrome in maintenance haemodialysis patients. *Nephrol Dial Transplant* 2003;18:217

38. Callaghan N. Restless legs syndrome in uremic neuropathy. *Neurology* 1966;16:359–61

39. Collado-Seidel V, Kohnen R, Samtleben W, *et al*. Clinical and biochemical findings in uremic patients with and without restless legs syndrome. *Am J Kidney Dis* 1998;31:324–8

40. Fukunishi I, Kitaoka T, Shirai T, Kino K. Facial paresthesias resembling restless legs syndrome in a patient on hemodialysis [letter]. *Nephron* 1998;79:485

41. Holley JL, Nespor S, Rault R. Characterizing sleep disorders in chronic hemodialysis patients. *ASAIO Trans* 1991;37:M456–7

42. Hui DS, Wong TY, Ko FW, *et al*. Prevalence of sleep disturbances in Chinese patients with end-stage renal failure on continuous ambulatory peritoneal dialysis. *Am J Kidney Dis*. [Computer file]. 2000;36:783–8

43. Hui DS, Wong TY, Li TS, *et al*. Prevalence of sleep disturbances in Chinese patients with end stage renal failure on maintenance hemodialysis. *Med Sci Monit* 2002;8:CR331–6

44. Huiqi Q, Shan L, Mingcai Q. Restless legs syndrome (RLS) in uremic patients is related to the frequency of hemodialysis sessions. *Nephron* 2000;86:540

45. Parker KP. Sleep disturbances in dialysis patients. *Sleep Med Rev* 2003;7:131–143

46. Pieta J, Millar T, Zacharias J, *et al*. Effect of pergolide on restless legs and leg movements in sleep in uremic patients. *Sleep* 1998;21:617–22

47. Roger SD, Harris DC, Stewart JH. Possible relation between restless legs and anaemia in renal dialysis patients [Letter]. *Lancet* 1991;337:1551

48. Sabbatini M, Minale B, Crispo A, *et al*. Insomnia in maintenance haemodialysis patients. *Nephrol Dial Transplant* 2002;17:852–6

49. Stepanski E, Faber M, Zorick F, *et al*. Sleep disorders in patients on continuous ambulatory peritoneal dialysis. *J Am Soc Nephrol* 1995;6:192–7

50. Walker SL, Fine A, Kryger MH. L-DOPA/carbidopa for nocturnal movement disorders in uremia. *Sleep* 1996;19:214–18

51. Virga G, Mastrosimone S, Amici G, *et al*. Symptoms in hemodialysis patients and their relationship with biochemical and demographic parameters. *Int J Artif Organs* 1998;21:788–93

52. Wetter TC, Stiasny K, Kohnen R, *et al*. Polysomnographic sleep measures in patients with uremic and idiopathic restless legs syndrome. *Mov Disord* 1998; 13:820–4

53. Winkelman JW, Chertow GM, Lazarus JM. Restless legs syndrome in end-stage renal disease. *Am J Kidney Dis* 1996;28:372–8

54. Read DJ, Feest TG, Nassim MA. Clonazepam: effective treatment for restless legs syndrome in uraemia. *Br Med J Clin Res Ed*. 1981;283:885–6

55. Tanaka K, Morimoto N, Tashiro N, *et al*. The features of psychological problems and their significance in patients on hemodialysis—with reference to social and somatic factors. *Clin Nephrol* 1999;51:161–76

56. Nielsen V.K. The peripheral nerve function in chronic renal failure. I. Clinical symptoms and signs *Acta Med Scand* 1971;190:105–11

57. Walker S, Fine A, Kryger MH. Sleep complaints are common in a dialysis unit. *Am J Kidney Dis* 1995;26:751–6

58. Bliwise D, Petta D, Seidel W, Dement W. Periodic leg movements during sleep in the elderly. *Arch Gerontol Geriatr* 1985;4:273–81

59. Bliwise DL, Ingham RH, Date ES, Dement WC. Nerve conduction and creatinine clearance in aged subjects with periodic movements in sleep. *J Gerontol* 1989;44:M164–7

60. Takaki J, Nishi T, Nangaku M, *et al*. Clinical and psychological aspects of restless legs syndrome in uremic patients on hemodialysis. *Am J Kidney Dis* 2003;41:833–9

61. Benz RL, Pressman MR, Peterson DD. Periodic limb movements of sleep index (PLMSI): a sensitive predictor of mortality in dialysis patients. 1994;5:433

62. Cirignotta F, Mondini S, Santoro A, *et al*. Reliability of a questionnaire screening restless legs syndrome in patients on chronic dialysis. *Am J Kidney Dis* 2002;40:302–6

63. Yasuda T, Nishimura A, Katsuki Y, Tsuji Y. Restless legs syndrome treated successfully by kidney transplantation—a case report. *Clin Transpl* 1986:138

64. Winkelmann J, Stautner A, Samtleben W, Trenkwalder C. Long-term course of restless legs syndrome in dialysis patients after kidney transplantation. *Mov Disord* 2002;17:1072–6

65. Janzen L, Rich JA, Vercaigne LM. An overview of levodopa in the management of restless legs syndrome in a dialysis population: pharmacokinetics, clinical trials, and complications of therapy. *Ann Pharmacother* 1999;33:86–92

66. Earley CJ, Connor JR, Beard JL, *et al*. Abnormalities in CSF concentrations of ferritin and transferrin in restless legs syndrome. *Neurology* 2000;54:1698–700

67. Allen RP, Barker PB, Wehrl F, Song HK, Earley CJ. MRI measurement of brain iron in patients with restless legs syndrome. *Neurology* 2001;56:263–5

68. Connor JR, Boyer PJ, Menzies SL, *et al*. Neuropathological examination suggests impaired brain iron acquisition in restless legs syndrome. *Neurology* 2003;61:304–9

69. Staedt J, Stoppe G, Kogler A, *et al*. Nocturnal myoclonus syndrome (periodic movements in sleep) related to central dopamine D2-receptor alteration. *Eur Arch Psychiatr Clin Neurosci* 1995;245:8–10

70. Trenkwalder C, Walters AS, Hening WA, *et al*. Positron emission tomographic studies in restless legs syndrome. *Mov Dis* 1999;14:141–5

71. Turjanski N, Lees AJ, Brooks DJ. Striatal dopaminergic function in restless legs syndrome: 18F-dopa and 11C-raclopride PET studies. *Neurology* 1999;52: 932–7

72. Nelson C, Erikson K, Pinero DJ, Beard JL. *In vivo* dopamine metabolism is altered in iron-deficient anemic rats. *J Nutr* 1997;127:2282–8

73. Ben-Shachar D, Finberg JP, Youdim MB. Effect of iron chelators on dopamine D2 receptors. *J Neurochem* 1985;45:999–1005

74. Ashkenazi R, Ben-Shachar D, Youdim MB. Nutritional iron and dopamine binding sites in the rat brain. *Pharmacol Biochem Behav* 1982;17 (Suppl 1):43–7

75. Ye Z, Connor JR. Identification of iron responsive genes by screening cDNA libraries from suppression subtractive hybridization with antisense probes from three iron conditions. *Nucleic Acids Res* 2000;28:1802–7

76. Jeng CJ, McCarroll SA, Martin TF, *et al*. Thy-1 is a component common to multiple populations of synaptic vesicles. *J Cell Biol* 1998;140:685–98

77. Shults CW, Kimber TA. Thy-1 immunoreactivity distinguishes patches/striosomes from matrix in the early postnatal striatum of the rat. *Brain Res Brain Res Dev* 1993;75:136–40

78. Glover J, Jacobs A. Activity pattern of iron-deficient rats. *BMJ* 1972;2:627–8

79. Youdim MB, Green AR, Bloomfield MR, *et al*. The effects of iron deficiency on brain biogenic monoamine biochemistry and function in rats. *Neuropharmacology* 1980;19:259–67

80. Norlander NB. Therapy in restless legs. *Acta Med Scand* 1953;143:453–7

81. Apenstrom G. Pica och restless legs vid jardbist. *Sven Lakartidn* 1964;61: 1174–7

82. Matthews WB. Iron deficiency and restless legs [Letter]. *BMJ* 1976;1:898

83. Ekbom KA. Restless legs: a report of 70 new cases. *Acta Med Scand Suppl* 1950; 246:64

84. Ekbom KA. Restless legs syndrome. *Neurology* 1960;10:868–73

85. Ondo WG, Vuong KD, Jankovic J. Exploring the relationship between Parkinson disease and restless legs syndrome. *Arch Neurol* 2002;59:421–4

86. O'Keeffe ST, Gavin K, Lavan JN. Iron status and restless legs syndrome in the elderly. *Age Ageing* 1994;23:200–3

87. Silber MH, Richardson JW. Multiple blood donations associated with iron deficiency in patients with restless legs syndrome. *Mayo Clin Proc* 2003;78:52–4

88. Sun ER, Chen CA, Ho G, Earley CJ, Allen RP. Iron and the restless legs syndrome. *Sleep* 1998;21:371–7

89. Aul EA, Davis BJ, Rodnitzky RL. The importance of formal serum iron studies in the assessment of restless legs syndrome. *Neurology* 1998;51:912

90. Berger K, von Eckardstein A, Trenkwalder C, *et al.* Iron metabolism and the risk of restless legs syndrome in an elderly general population—the MEMO-Study. *J Neurol* 2002;249:1195–9

91. Ondo W, Tan EK, Mansoor J. Rheumatologic serologies in secondary restless legs syndrome. *Mov Disord* 2000;15:321–3

92. Earley CJ, Allen RP, Beard JL, Connor JR. Insight into the pathophysiology of restless legs syndrome. *J Neurosci Res* 2000;62:623–8

93. O'Keeffe ST, Noel J, Lavan JN. Restless legs syndrome in the elderly. *Postgrad Med J* 1993;69:701–3

94. Davis BJ, Rajput A, Rajput ML, *et al.* A randomized, double-blind placebo-controlled trial of iron in restless legs syndrome. *Eur Neurol* 2000;43:70–5

95. Earley CJ, Heckler D, allen RP. IV Iron treatment for the restless legs syndrome (RLS). *Sleep* 2001;24 (Suppl):A359

96. Goodman JD, Brodie C, Ayida GA. Restless leg syndrome in pregnancy. *BMJ* 1988;297:1101–2

97. Manconi M, Govoni V, Cesnik E, *et al.* Epidemiology of restless legs syndrome in a population of 606 pregnant women. *Sleep* 2003;26 (Abstr Suppl): A300–A301

98. Lee KA, Zaffke ME, Baratte-Beebe K. Restless legs syndrome and sleep disturbance during pregnancy: the role of folate and iron. *J Womens Health Gend Based Med* 2001;10:335–41

99. Botez MI, Lambert B. Folate deficiency and restless-legs syndrome in pregnancy [Letter]. *N Engl J Med* 1977;297:670

100. Winkelmann J, Wetter TC, Collado-Seidel V, *et al.* Clinical characteristics and frequency of the hereditary restless legs syndrome in a population of 300 patients. *Sleep* 2000;23:597–602

101. Ruottinen HM, Partinen M, Hublin C, *et al*. An FDOPA PET study in patients with periodic limb movement disorder and restless legs syndrome. *Neurology* 2000;54:502–4

102. Wetter TC, Collado-Seidel V, Pollmacher T, *et al*. Sleep and periodic leg movement patterns in drug-free patients with Parkinson's disease and multiple system atrophy. *Sleep* 2000;23:361–7

103. Horiguchi J, Inami Y, Nishimatsu O, *et al*. [Sleep-wake complaints in Parkinson's disease]. *Rinsho Shinkeigaku* 1990;30:214–16

104. Banno K, Delaive K, Walld R, Kryger M. Restless legs syndrome in 218 patients: associated disorders. *Sleep Med* 2000;1:221–9

105. Paulson G. Is restless legs a prodrome to Parkinson's disease. *Mov Disord* (Suppl 1) 1997;12:68

106. Lang AE. Restless legs syndrome and Parkinson's disease: insights into pathophysiology. *Clin Neuropharmacol* 1987;10:476–8

107. Krishnan PR, Bhatia M, Behari M. Restless legs syndrome in Parkinson's disease: A case-controlled study. *Mov Disord* 2003;18:181–5

108. Tan EK, Lum SY, Wong MC. Restless legs syndrome in Parkinson's disease. *J Neurol Sci* 2002;196:33–6

109. Fazzini E, Diaz R, Fahn S. Restless legs in Parkinson's disease-clinical evidence for underactivity of catecholamine neurotransmission. 1989 [Abstract];26:142

110. Higgins JJ, Loveless JM, Jankovic J, Patel PI. Evidence that a gene for essential tremor maps to chromosome 2p in four families. *Mov Disord* 1998;13:972–7

111. Larner AJ, Allen CM. Hereditary essential tremor and restless legs syndrome [Letter]. *Postgraduate Med J* 1997;73:254

112. Abele M, Burk K, Laccone F, *et al*. Restless legs syndrome in spinocerebellar ataxia types 1, 2, and 3. *J Neurol* 2001;248:311–14

113. Schols L, Haan J, Riess O, *et al*. Sleep disturbance in spinocerebellar ataxias: is the SCA3 mutation a cause of restless legs syndrome? *Neurology* 1998;51:1603–7

114. van Alfen N, Sinke RJ, Zwarts MJ, *et al*. Intermediate CAG repeat lengths (53,54) for MJD/SCA3 are associated with an abnormal phenotype. *Ann Neurol* 2001;49:805–7

115. Reynolds G, Blake DR, Pall HS, Williams A. Restless leg syndrome and rheumatoid arthritis. *Br Med J Clin Res Ed*. 1986;292:659–60

116. Salih AM, Gray RE, Mills KR, Webley M. A clinical, serological and neurophysiological study of restless legs syndrome in rheumatoid arthritis. *Br J Rheumatol* 1994;33:60–3

117. Gudbjornsson B, Broman JE, Hetta J, Hallgren R. Sleep disturbances in patients with primary Sjogren's syndrome. *Br J Rheumatol* 1993;32:1072–6

118. Yunus MB, Aldag JC. Restless legs syndrome and leg cramps in fibromyalgia syndrome: a controlled study. *BMJ* 1996;312:1339

119. Moldofsky H. Management of sleep disorders in fibromyalgia. *Rheum Dis Clin North Am* 2002;28:353–65

120. Schonbrunn E, Riemann D, Hohagen F, Berger M. Restless legs und Schlafapnoesyndrom—zufallige Koinzidenz oder kausale Beziehung? *Nervenarzt* 1990;61:306–11

121. Coccagna G, Lugaresi E. Restless legs syndrome and nocturnal myoclonus. *Int J Neurol* 1981;15:77–87

122. Evers S, Stogbauer F. Genetic association of Huntington's disease and restless legs syndrome? A family report. *Mov Disord* 2003;18:226–8

123. Schlienger JL. Syndrome des membres inferieurs impatients du a une hypothyroidie moderee. *Presse Medicale* 1985;14:791

124. Spillane JD. Restless legs syndrome in chronic pulmonary disease. *BMJ* 1970;4:796–8

125. Stein JA, Tschudy DP. Acute intermittent porphyria. A clinical and biochemical study of 46 patients. *Medicine* 1970;49:1–16

126. Ekbom KA. Restless legs syndrome after partial gastrectomy. *Acta Neurol Scand* 1966;42:79–84

127. Balmer A, Limoni C. Klinische, plazebokontrollierte Doppelblindprufung von Venoruton bei der Behandlung der chronisch-venosen Insuffizienz. Die Bedeutung der Patientenauswahl. *Vasa* 1980;9:76–82

128. McEwan AJ, McArdle CS. Effect of hydroxyethylrutosides on blood oxygen levels and venous insufficiency symptoms in varicose veins. *BMJ* 1971;2:138–41

129. Harvey JC. Cholesterol crystal microembolization: a cause of the restless leg syndrome. *South Med J* 1976;69:269–72

130. Muller N, Voderholzer U, Kurtz G, Straube A. Tourette's syndrome associated with restless legs syndrome and akathisia in a family. *Acta Neurol Scand* 1994;89:429–32

131. Lugaresi E, Cirignotta F, Coccagna G, Montagna P. Nocturnal myoclonus and restless legs syndrome. *Adv Neurol* 1986;43:295–307

132. Akpinar S. Restless legs syndrome treatment with dopaminergic drugs. *Clin Neuropharmacol* 1987;10:69–79

133. Metcalfe RA, MacDermott N, Chalmers RJ. Restless red legs: an association of the restless legs syndrome with arborizing telangiectasia of the lower limbs. *J Neurol Neurosurg Psychiatr* 1986;49:820–3

134. Winkelmann J, Schadrack J, Wetter TC, *et al*. Opioid and dopamine antagonist drug challenges in untreated restless legs syndrome. Sleep Med 2001;2:57–61

135. Wetter TC, Brunner J, Bronisch T. Restless legs syndrome probably induced by risperidone treatment. *Pharmacopsychiatry* 2002;35:109–11

136. Kraus T, Schuld A, Pollmacher T. Periodic leg movements in sleep and restless legs syndrome probably caused by olanzapine [Letter]. *J Clin Psychopharmacol* 1999;19:478–9

137. Chen JT, Garcia PA, Alldredge BK. Zonisamide-induced restless legs syndrome. *Neurology* 2003;60:147

138. Bahk WM, Pae CU, Chae JH, *et al*. Mirtazapine may have the propensity for developing a restless legs syndrome? A case report. *Psychiatry Clin Neurosci* 2002;56:209–10

139. Teive HA, Quadros Ad A, Barros FC, Werneck LC. Worsening of autosomal dominant restless legs syndrome after use of mirtazapine: case report. *Arq Neuropsiquiatr* 2002;60:1025–9

140. Markkula J, Lauerma H. Mianserin and restless legs. *Int Clin Psychopharmacol* 1997;12:53–8

141. Sanz-Fuentenebro FJ, Huidobro A, Tejadas-Rivas A. Restless legs syndrome and paroxetine. *Acta Psychiatr Scand* 1996;94:482–4

142. Hargrave R, Beckley DJ. Restless leg syndrome exacerbated by sertraline [Letter]. *Psychosomatics* 1998;39:177–8

143. Dimmitt SB, Riley GJ. Selective serotonin receptor uptake inhibitors can reduce restless legs symptoms. *Arch Intern Med* 2000;160:712

144. Heiman EM, Christie M. Lithium-aggravated nocturnal myoclonus and restless legs syndrome [Letter]. *Am J Psychiatry* 1986;143:1191–2

145. Terao T, Terao M, Yoshimura R, Abe K. Restless legs syndrome induced by lithium. *Biol Psychiatry* 1991;30:1167–70

146. Bastani B, Westervelt FB. Effectiveness of clonidine in alleviating the symptoms of 'restless legs' [Letter]. *Am J Kidney Dis* 1987;10:326

Restless legs syndrome: differential diagnosis and treatment

W. Tse, W. Koller and C. W. Olanow

INTRODUCTION

Restless legs syndrome (RLS) is a disorder characterized by a sensation of unpleasant paresthesias occurring mainly in the legs associated with an irresistible desire to move the affected extremities. Symptoms are typically alleviated by movement and tend to occur predominantly while at rest during the evening hours, but may also occur during the day. These disagreeable sensations and movements may lead to nocturnal insomnia and chronic sleep deprivation with excessive daytime sleepiness and impaired quality of life. The condition is frequently unrecognized or misdiagnosed because patients may have difficulty describing the sensation (often using terms such as itchy, creepy, or crawly) and may be unaware that they suffer chronic sleepiness. The syndrome was first described in 1672 by Sir Thomas Willis as a night-time 'unquietness' of the limbs that interfered with sleep[1,2]. Karl A. Ekbom, a Swedish neurologist and surgeon, published a comprehensive account of this syndrome in 1945 and termed it 'restless legs'[3]. Lugaresi and colleagues subsequently used polysomnographic monitoring to document the involuntary leg movements seen in 87.8% of patients with RLS and termed them periodic limb movements of sleep (PLMS)[4]. PLMS have subsequently been described in several other sleep disorders and neurologic diseases[5], including narcolepsy[6,7], obstructive sleep apnea[8] and Parkinson's disease[9].

The prevalence estimates for RLS have been reported to range between 5 and 15% in adult white populations[10–12]. Ulfberg and co-workers studied a population of 4000 Swedish men between the ages of 18 and 64 years, and discovered a mean prevalence of 5.8%, with the oldest age group (55–64 years) having a prevalence of more than 10%[13]. The MEMO study, a population-based survey of an elderly population, reported a higher prevalence of RLS in women, with a mean prevalence of 9.8%[14]. This study also demonstrated that RLS symptoms are associated with impaired health status and decreased mental and general health scores. Whereas it is agreed that RLS is a common condition, the frequency of disabling symptoms that require treatment remains to be determined.

Although RLS is often thought to be a condition of the middle-aged and elderly population, recent studies show that symptoms frequently appear in childhood and adolescence[15]. Indeed, retrospective assessments indicate that the onset of RLS occurred before the age of 20 years in as many as 43% of adult cases[16,17]. On the other hand, older patients complain more about RLS symptoms, suggesting that the disease is progressive and chronic condition. In many female patients, RLS symptoms manifest initially during pregnancy, remit and then reappear in later years[18].

Differential diagnosis of RLS (Table 7.1)

The differential diagnosis of RLS is broad and encompasses a large number of motor and sensory disorders (Table 7.1). Most commonly, RLS may be confused with polyneuropathy. Both disorders may present with paresthesias affecting the distal legs. It is also possible that the two disorders can coexist in the same patient[19]. Typically, patients with peripheral neuropathy in the absence of RLS do not experience worsening at rest with relief by

Table 7.1   Differential diagnosis of RLS

Motor syndromes
Akathisia
Nocturnal leg cramps
Positional discomfort
Painful leg moving toes
Myoclonus of sleep
    hypnic myoclonus (sleep starts)
    fragmentory myoclonus
    spinal myoclonus
Muscle pain fasciculation syndrome
Hypotensive akathisia

Sensory syndrome
Polyneuropathy
Vascular diseases of legs
    claudication
    venous stasis
Causalgia-dystonia syndrome

Others (as a consquence of RLS)
Insomnia
Affective disorders

activity, and symptoms do not worsen at night. Testing with polysomnography may be helpful in differentiating the two conditions, as the finding of PLMS on sleep studies is supportive of the diagnosis of RLS.

A rare syndrome of pain in the feet or lower limbs associated with spontaneous movements of the toes is known as the 'painful leg and moving toes' syndrome. Flexion and extension movements of the toes are found on examination. In contrast to RLS, patients with this syndrome do not achieve relief of their painful sensations with movements and the involuntary movements tend to disappear in sleep[20–22].

Akathisia can occur spontaneously or secondary to the use of dopamine receptor blocking agents. Features can include motor restlessness and sleep disturbances that can be confused with RLS[23]. However, PLM are not common in akathisia[24], restlessness not referable to the extremities is typical, paresthesias are not usually present and RLS symptoms are more likely to be exacerbated at night and at rest[25]. In addition, dopaminergic drugs may worsen or trigger akathisia particularly in some cases of parkinsonism[26], whereas they usually ameliorate the symptoms of RLS.

Nocturnal leg cramps may present with painful sensations in the legs that can be confused with the abnormal sensations associated with RLS. Nocturnal muscle cramps usually involve painful sustained contractions of the calf muscles (gastrocnemius or soleus) and are particularly common in the elderly or during pregnancy. Relief of muscle cramps can sometimes be achieved by dorsiflexion maneuvers that stretch the contracted muscles. Quinine and vitamin E are also effective treatments[27–29].

Myoclonus can also be confused with RLS. Myoclonus is an involuntary, brief muscle contraction that produces a visible twitch of a body segment. Several types of myoclonus have been described in sleep. Hypnic myoclonus, or sleep starts, can be observed in normal individuals during the transition from wakefulness to sleep[30]. Fragmentary myoclonus consists of asynchronous, twitch-like jerks that occur mainly in the hands and face, characteristically during REM sleep[31]. Myoclonus of spinal origin has also been described in which the myoclonus is limited to muscles innervated by a few adjacent spinal segments, and is usually due to local spinal pathology. Abnormal activity in the long propriospinal pathways has been reported to generate a complex and extensive form of spinal myoclonus, with repetitive non-rhythmic flexor jerks of the neck, trunk, both hips and knees. Spinal myoclonus, like PLMS, can also persist in sleep[32–34]. Patients with spinal cord lesions will often have localizing neurologic signs on examination, such as spasticity, leg weakness or a sensory impairment at that level.

Another unusual syndrome that can be confused with RLS is the muscular pain-fasciculation syndrome which is a chronic neuromuscular condition consisting of muscular aching, burning pain, cramps, fasciculations and occasional paresthesias. This disorder usually affects the legs and, less commonly, the girdle, trunk and arm muscles. In contrast to RLS, symptoms are relieved rather than precipitated by rest. In addition, patients with idiopathic RLS do not typically have fasciculations[35,36]. The pathogenesis of this disorder is unclear, but neurophysiologic studies provide evidence of axonal neuropathy.

Another condition is hypotensive akathisia, where patients with autonomic failure manifest voluntary, transiently suppressible leg movements in the sitting position. The movements represent an adaptive mechanism to reduce symptomatic declines in blood pressure in the sitting position[37]. Unlike RLS, limb restlessness occurs only while the patient is in the sitting position and resolves when the patient is supine. Sleep in these cases is undisturbed and orthostatic hypotension is not a feature of RLS.

Vascular disease of the legs may also present with painful leg sensations. However, patients with vascular claudication usually experience worsening of leg pains with walking and improvement with rest. There may also be physical signs on examination to suggest arterial or venous disease such as leg edema, venous stasis skin changes or decreased pulses.

Another syndrome consists of burning pain with hyperpathia as well as vasomotor, sudomotor and trophic changes, initially in one limb[38]. Patients may be diagnosed as having a 'causalgia–dystonia' syndrome because they present with a painful, fixed, focal dystonia. The causalgia and dystonia in these patients may spread beyond the original affected site to involve other extremities. All investigations are normal in these patients and it is unclear whether the syndrome represents a true neurologic disease or is psychogenic in origin.

Since RLS can present primarily as insomnia or a sleep disturbance, it is likely that some patients with RLS are mistakenly diagnosed as being depressed. There may, therefore, be a tendency to ascribe a psychological etiology to a sleep disturbance without sufficiently searching for an organic cause. It is important to consider that RLS can be disguised as an affective disorder. A complete sleep history and polysomnography are necessary to establish the diagnosis[39–41].

TREATMENT OF RESTLESS LEGS SYNDROME

Assessment

Since RLS is frequently misdiagnosed or under-recognized, the first step towards proper treatment of patients with RLS is accurate diagnosis of the condition[42,43]. Physicians should take special care to consider the diagnosis of RLS in patients in whom sleep disturbances represent the initial presenting symptom. Although not required for diagnosis, the sleep disturbances associated with RLS can be severely disabling and represent the primary morbidity[44]. The diagnosis of RLS is based mainly on the patient's history, assessing for the (IRLSSG) criteria. Neurologic examination is typically normal and should be performed to rule out potentially treatable illnesses that may cause or exacerbate secondary RLS. Clinical and physiologic examination should, in particular, be directed towards seeking evidence of peripheral nerve or spinal dysfunction. Blood tests are done primarily to screen for anemia, iron storage dysfunction, diabetes and renal insufficiency. It should be noted that iron deficiency may be present in the absence of anemia. Thus, iron status, as indicated by serum ferritin level and iron saturation, should be assessed as patients may benefit from iron supplementation when the serum ferritin level is less than 50 ng/ml. Other tests to evaluate RLS can include actigraphy, polysomnographic studies, and the Suggested Immobilization Test (SIT) (see Chapter 9). In actigraphy, muscle activity is monitored with a small portable meter worn at the ankle (see Chapter 9). Actigraphic devices do not differentiate between PLM and other movements. Polysomnography is a useful adjunctive test that can detect PLMS by EMG recordings from the tibialis anterior muscle. A PLM index (number of PLMS) of greater than 5 during one night of sleep is considered pathologic and is consistent with the diagnosis of RLS. The frequency of PLMS is used as a measure of disease severity and can be used to follow treatment response. Polysomnography is also useful to rule out other sleep disorders such as sleep apnea and to evaluate the contribution of PLMS to sleep disruption. SIT was developed to quantify PLMs in wakefulness. Patients are asked to remain immobile while EMG recordings from tibialis anterior muscles indicate leg movements occurring during the test. However, the sensitivity of the SIT has not been studied in large numbers of RLS patients.

Treatment

Initial therapy of RLS is based on the severity of symptoms and their impact on the patient's well-being[45]. The frequency with which RLS symptoms cause meaningful disability is not known, but it is thought that 20–25% of RLS patients have symptoms severe enough to warrant pharmacologic treatment. Non-pharmacologic treatments for RLS may suffice for patients with mild RLS (Table 7.2). For some, mild walking or movement of the

Table 7.2 *Non-pharmacologic measures useful for the treatment of RLS*

Sleep hygiene:
    avoiding tea/coffee/alcohol before bedtime
    avoiding disturbing reading material
    advising sleeping late and rising late
    cool comfortable sleeping environment
Avoid RLS-inducing drugs
Treat iron deficiency if present
During an attack of RLS the following may help:
    walking and stretching
    relaxation exercises (biofeedback or yoga)
    engaging in discussion to distract mind
    massaging affected limbs

affected limb may alleviate symptoms. Hot or cold baths or performing tasks requiring concentration may also help some patients. Improvement of sleep hygiene is important, and should include regular sleeping hours and avoidance of stimulants such as caffeine prior to bedtime. Secondary causes of RLS due to reversible medical conditions should be identified and treated. Symptoms due to physiologic conditions such as pregnancy will often remit spontaneously after delivery. Patients with iron deficiency should be supplemented with iron. Improvement in RLS symptoms has also been described after pallidotomy[46]. Pharmacologic treatment of RLS has largely focused on the use of four classes of drugs: dopaminergic, opioids, benzodiazepines and anticonvulsants (Table 7.3).

Dopaminergic medications

Levodopa Dopaminergic agents are the best studied and widely used class of medications for the treatment of RLS and are generally considered the treatment of choice. The efficacy of levodopa combined with a dopa decarboxylase inhibitor (e.g. carbidopa or benserazide) was first demonstrated in an open label trial[47]. Subsequently, levodopa has been studied in a large number of double-blind placebo-controlled trials. Doses studied range from 50 to 600 mg/day, given either at night or in divided doses. In these studies, levodopa has been shown to be well tolerated and to result in a significant reduction in PLMS frequency and improvement in nocturnal symptoms and quality of sleep for patients with both primary and secondary RLS[48-50]. Levodopa's rapid onset of action has been demonstrated in a double-blind crossover trial, in which symptom relief was achieved with administration of a single bedtime dose of levodopa/benserazide, 25/100 mg or 50/200 mg, respectively, with full efficacy achieved within the first few days of therapy. Levodopa therapy had significantly superior efficacy to placebo during the first half of the night (hours 1 to 4) but not during the second half of the night (hour 5 to waking), demonstrating levodopa's relatively short duration of action[51]. A long-term follow-up study showed the sustained benefits of levodopa therapy in RLS over 2 years, although increased dosing was needed in some patients[52].

Two important complications of long-term levodopa therapy of RLS are rebound and augmentation. The 'end-of-dose rebound effect' consists of a recurrence of RLS symptoms in the latter half of the night or early morning after nocturnal levodopa administration[53]. This phenomenon is typically seen with use of the regular release form of levodopa, suggesting that it may be due to a wearing-off effect. Rebound effects may be improved by using a sustained release formulation of levodopa at bedtime or by additional daytime dosing prior to symptom recurrence. In a retrospective study 91.5% of RLS patients reported an initial good response to levodopa therapy. At 6 months, 70% had continued benefit from a single bedtime levodopa dose (mean 160 mg), but 46% of these required a second dose later in the night due to the reappearance of symptoms[54]. A subsequent double-blind study showed that in patients randomized to a combination of standard levodopa (100–200 mg), the combination and slow-release levodopa (100–200 mg) was more effective than standard levodopa alone in improving RLS symptoms and decreasing periodic limb movement frequency[55]. Augmentation refers to a shifting to an earlier time of onset of RLS symptoms after long-term levodopa treatment – in the early evening or during the daytime.

Patients with augmentation may also experience an intensification of their symptoms and the emergence of symptoms in other limbs. This phenomenon has been described in more than 80% of RLS patients after 2 months of levodopa treatment. High levodopa dosages of more than 200 mg/day, the presence of RLS symptoms before 6 pm prior to starting treatment, and severe RLS symptoms have all been correlated with the development of augmentation[56]. In comparison, augmentation has been reported in only 20–30% of patients on dopamine agonists[57,58]. Thus, the daily levodopa dose should be kept to a maximum of 400 mg/day and dopamine agonists should be used in patients who develop augmentation on levodopa. It has been suggested that the lower incidence of augmentation reported with dopamine agonists may be due to the relatively low doses employed and the shorter treatment duration in various clinical trials, and

Table 7.3 Drugs used to treat restless legs syndrome (modified from Chaudhuri KR and Earley CJ)

Drug class	Maximum recommended doses	Comments
Levodopa (with carbidopa or benserazide)	100–600 mg/day in evening or divided doses Initial dose: 50 mg	Long-term complications include augmentation (reported in 80% of patients) and rebound (reported in 20% of patients)
Dopamine agonists		
Bromocriptine	2.5–7.5 mg/day Initial dose 2.5 mg	Demonstrated equivalent effect to levodopa in one study but levodopa was better tolerated
Pergolide	0.05–0.75 mg/day, in evening or divided doses Initial dose: 0.05 mg	As an ergot derivative, is associated with rare side-effects of pleuropulmonary and retroperitoneal fibrosis, erythromelalgia Dopaminergic side-effects, i.e. nausea, hypotension, nasal stuffiness, typically warrant slow titration upwards Augmentation has been reported in 20–30% of patients
Pramipexole	0.25–1.5 mg/day, in evening or divided doses	Lower risk of ergot-related side-effects, but may have increased risk of sedation and edema compared with older ergot agents. Augmentation reported in 32% of patients
Ropinirole	0.25–4 mg/day, in evening or divided doses	Side-effects similar to pramipexole. No augmentation reported.
Cabergoline	2.1 mg/day mean dose, single evening dose	Longest-acting dopamine agonist and can be given once a day. May be effective for patients with augmentation

Continued

Table 7.3 Continued

Drug class	Maximum recommended doses	Comments
Opiates		
Propoxyphene	100–600 mg/day, in evening or divided doses. Initial dose: 100–200 mg	Side-effects include sedation, dependence and constipation. May be effective in painful RLS. No augmentation reported
Oxycodone	20–30 mg/day, in evening or divided doses. Initial dose: 5 mg	Same side-effect profile as propoxyphene
Antiepileptic medications		
Gabapentin	1500–3600 mg/day in divided doses. Initial dose: 300 mg	Side-effects include sedation, dizziness. May be effective in painful RLS
Carbamazepine	100–300 mg/day, in divided doses. Initial dose: 100 mg	Has been shown to improve subjective RLS symptoms but not PLMS symptoms
Benzodiazepines		
Clonazepam	0.25–2 mg at bedtime	Side-effects include sedation and tolerance. May be useful in patients with insomnia
Other medications		
Iron	200 mg po TID*	Improvement noted in patients with iron deficiency anemia, i.e. with ferritin levels < 45 ng/ml
Clonidine	0.5–0.9 mg/day	Associated with significant side-effects of depression, sedation, headache, hypotension

*po TID, orally three times daily

that higher doses of dopamine agonists and long-term use may result in augmentation rates similar to levodopa[59].

Dopamine agonists Bromocriptine was the first dopamine receptor agonist studied for the treatment of RLS. A double-blind placebo-controlled trial using a mean dose of 7.5 mg given as an evening dose provided a significant decrease in the number of PLMS[60]. A comparison of levodopa and bromocriptine showed equivalent subjective improvement with both medications, but levodopa was better tolerated. Pergolide, a long-acting ergot dopamine agonist, has been the most extensively studied drug in the treatment of RLS (summarized in reference 61). In general, these studies demonstrate significant benefits of pergolide on RLS symptoms. One double-blind placebo-controlled study showed that a mean pergolide dosage of 0.5 mg was efficacious in reducing the number of PLMS and improving subjective sleep quality[62]. Formal comparisons among the different dopamine agonists have not been performed, but several studies have compared pergolide to levodopa. In one series of 51 patients treated initially with levodopa, 73% of the 26 patients who were switched to pergolide for unsatisfactory symptom control reported improvement with pergolide[63]. Patients with PLMS responded best to levodopa, whereas those with the most severe RLS symptoms responded best to pergolide. Another prospective study similarly demonstrated the efficacy of pergolide in patients considered to be levodopa failures due to the development of augmentation[64]. However, 15% of patients in this study discontinued pergolide due to dopaminergic side-effects such as nausea, nasal stuffiness and dizziness. A randomized crossover trial of 0.125 mg of pergolide vs. 250 mg of levodopa/carbidopa demonstrated that pergolide was not only more effective in relieving RLS symptoms, but also increased total sleep time[65]. In a 2-year study, 45% of RLS patients treated with a median dose of 0.18 mg of pergolide reported complete to near-complete relief of symptoms, while an additional 50% experienced moderate relief[57]. Side-effects, including nausea, dizziness, insomnia, and constipation, occurred in 60% of patients and led to discontinuation in 25%. Augmentation occurred in 27% of patients, although it was usually mild and well-controlled with an additional dose of pergolide. It may be that the apparent efficacy of pergolide over levodopa is related to its longer half-life (29 hours for pergolide versus 1–3 hours for levodopa). Disadvantages of pergolide include frequent side-effects and the necessity for a long titration period to the optimal therapeutic dosage[62].

In an attempt to avoid the side-effects associated with ergoline derivatives, the non-ergot dopamine agonists pramipexole and ropinirole have recently been evaluated for the treatment of RLS. A double-blind, randomized crossover trial demonstrated that pramipexole in doses of 0.375 mg to 0.75 mg/day provided significant subjective improvement in RLS symptoms with reduced PLMS[66]. However, sleep parameters such as total sleep time, number of awakenings, and sleep efficiency were unchanged. Follow-up studies demonstrate long-term efficacy of pramipexole over a 7.8-month treatment period, in single bedtime doses ranging from 0.25 mg to 0.75 mg[67]. In an open-label study, pramipexole provided effective treatment for patients who demonstrated treatment resistance to other dopaminergic agents due to the development of daytime augmentation[68]. Pramipexole is well tolerated, with mild, transient side-effects of nausea, dizziness and daytime fatigue mostly at the initiation of treatment, which usually resolve with reduction in dose and do not necessitate discontinuation of the medication. Augmentation develops in approximately 5–10% of patients who have received pramipexole for at least 6 months, and is thought to be more likely to occur in patients with secondary RLS than in those with idiopathic RLS and in those with sub-optimal therapeutic doses[69,70]. More recent studies suggest that augmentation may be more common than originally supposed. In a retrospective chart review of 50 RLS patients treated with pramipexole, 18% developed augmentation after a mean duration of 8.5 months[71]. Another retrospective study found augmentation in 32% of 59 patients after a mean of 8.8 months of treatment[72]. This problem was readily managed by earlier administration of pramipexole and only rarely led to discontinuation of the treatment. Tolerance also developed in 46% of pramipexole-treated patients. However, the majority of these patients had previously experienced augmentation or tolerance on levodopa and many of the patients were on other medications for RLS during pramipexole treatment. Controlled trials will need to be carried out to further evaluate the long-term risk of augmentation or tolerance with pramipexole.

Ropinirole is another non-ergot dopamine agonist that has recently been studied for RLS. An initial open-label trial involving 16 patients demonstrated significant improvement in IRLSSG questionnaire scores after treatment with ropinirole at a mean daily dose of 2.8 mg[73]. Thirteen patients completed the study and reported a 58.7% improvement in questionnaire scores. Three patients did not complete the study because of adverse events, such as rash and anxiety. Sleep laboratory studies further demonstrated that ropinirole in evening doses of 0.5 mg was associated with improvement in sleep architecture with increased total sleep time and efficiency[74]. Most recently, the TREAT RLS 1 Study, a randomized placebo-controlled study, demonstrated that ropinirole at single doses of up to 4 mg/day was significantly more effective than placebo in alleviating RLS symptomatology, improving sleep quantity and adequacy, reducing sleep disturbance and daytime somnolence, and improving health-related quality of life[75]. The efficacy of ropinirole was apparent within 1 week of treatment. It is anticipated that ropinirole will soon receive the first FDA approval as treatment for RLS.

Cabergoline is the longest-acting dopamine agonist with a biological half-life of 65 hours. Cabergoline was studied in an open-label trial of nine patients who had previously experienced augmentation on levodopa. Improvement in RLS symptoms and a decrease in the number of PLMS were recorded in a 12-week open-label study with a mean dose of 2.1 mg/day[76]. These results were confirmed in a placebo-controlled, double-blind trial comparing 0.5–2 mg of cabergoline with placebo[77]. In the UK, cabergoline is widely used for the treatment of RLS and recent studies have suggsted that it is well tolerated, with little risk of augmentation, rebound or fibrotic side-effects after 6 years of follow-up[78,79].

Rotigotine is a novel dopamine agonist that is administered via a trans-dermal patch. A dose-dependent reduction in RLS severity was observed in a double-blind, placebo-controlled pilot study[80]. Overnight nocturnal infusion of apomorphine, a subcutaneous dopamine agonist, has also been shown to be effective in reducing nocturnal discomfort, with improved pain and spasm scores in two RLS patients[81].

Benzodiazepines Clinical experience suggests that benzodiazepines are of some value in the treatment of RLS, however, the results of double-blind studies have been mixed. Clonazepam is the most widely studied benzo-diazepine, and in a parallel-design study doses ranging from 0.5 to 2 mg were associated with a significant decrease in PLMS[82]. The direct effects of benzodiazepines on RLS are difficult to ascertain, however, as the medications may have confounding effects on sleep variables because of their strong sedating properties. In addition, significant side-effects may occur with benzodiazepines, including daytime sleepiness, confusion and respiratory depression, which may limit their use, particularly in elderly patients. Augmentation has not been reported, although this has not been formally studied.

Antiepileptic medications Several anti-convulsant medications have been shown to be useful in the treatment of RLS. In a double-blind study, carba-mazepine was more effective than placebo in improving RLS symptoms and sleep at doses of 100–300 mg/day; however, many patients in the carbamazepine arm experienced side-effects and dropped out of the study[83]. In another study, PLMS and PLMS-associated arousals were not reduced by carbamazepine treatment[84]. Gabapentin has been evaluated in open-label trials as well as in a 6-week, double-blind, cross over study. In the double-blind study, patients were initiated on gabapentin at a dose of 600 mg/day, which was increased as needed to control symptoms up to a maximum of 2400 mg/day. At a mean dose of 1855 mg, gabapentin improved subjective RLS symptoms and sleep outcomes and significantly reduced the PLMS index. Patients with higher pain scores on a visual pain analogue scale (PAS) sustained the most benefit[85]. Gabapentin has been compared with ropinirole in an open clinical trial. Patients were treated with an initial dose of either 300 mg of gabapentin or 0.5 mg of ropinirole with titration upwards until symptom relief was achieved. A mean gabapentin dosage of 800 mg and a mean ropinirole dosage of 0.78 mg were well tolerated and provided comparable treatment of the PLMS and sensorimotor symptoms of RLS[86]. Valproate has also been shown to be effective in the treatment of the sleep disturbance of PLMD in an open-label trial[87]. In general, anti-epileptic medications appear to have a more limited therapeutic effect compared with dopaminergic agents. They may be considered in the treatment of RLS when dopaminergic agents fail to provide sufficient benefit and may be particularly useful in cases of RLS with a significant pain component.

Opioid medications

Opioids have been used for the treatment of RLS since the 17th century, when Willis described improvement with the use of laudanum. Two double-blind, randomized placebo-controlled trials have been carried out with oxycodone and propoxyphene. Oxycodone, at a mean daily dose of 15.9 mg, was shown to be effective for the treatment of RLS symptoms and sleep disturbances, with evidence of decreased PLMS and associated arousals, and improved sleep efficiency[88].

Propoxyphene in doses of up to 300 mg was associated with an improvement in RLS subjective symptoms but levodopa was more effective in reducing periodic limb movements[89,90].

Opioid medications can thus be considered in patients with a refractory response to dopaminergic agents. Side-effects of constipation and nausea as well as concern about addiction limit their usefulness. However, there has been little evidence for the development of tolerance or addiction in limited series[91].

Other medications

Treatment of iron deficiency anemia (as manifested by a ferritin level less than 50 ng/ml) with iron supplementation has been shown to improve or resolve RLS symptoms[92].

One open-label trial demonstrated that supplementation with oral iron, 200 mg three times a day, improved symptoms maximally in patients with the lowest ferritin levels (<18 ng/ml)[93].The benefits of oral iron treatment, when present, are noted to occur after several weeks or months of treatment[94]. In patients with normal to high ferritin levels, one double-blind, placebo-controlled trial failed to show benefit of oral iron therapy[95], but intravenous iron therapy was reported to improve RLS symptoms in 21 of 22 patients with normal serum iron levels[96].

Further studies to clarify the role of iron in the treatment of RLS are warranted.

There are anecdotal reports indicating that propranolol is beneficial in RLS. Clonidine, an adrenergic agonist, has been shown in a randomized, double-blind, placebo-controlled study to be effective in treating the symptoms of RLS, but did not decrease the number of PLMS[97]. Side-effects were frequent but generally mild, and included dry mouth, sleepiness, decreased cognition and headache. Clonidine is generally regarded as second-line therapy for the treatment of RLS. Baclofen was tested in a study that included polysomnography and was found to reduce PLMS amplitude as well as resultant sleep disruptions due to PLMS-related arousals, but it increased the total number of PLMS[98]. It has not been formally studied for the treatment of RLS. Anecdotal benefits in RLS have also been reported for a number of other medications including vitamin B_{12}, vitamin E, folic acid and epidural morphine. One case report has described the successful use of entacapone to increase the duration of symptom relief in a patient with RLS treated with levodopa/carbidopa[99].

Treatment guidelines for RLS

In 1999, the American Academy of Sleep Medicine developed practice guidelines for the treatment of RLS and PLMD, based on a review of the medical literature[45]. They recommend limiting pharmacologic treatment to RLS patients who met specific diagnostic criteria based on history, symptom severity and impact on well-being. In these patients, benefit from medications must be weighed individually against the potential for side-effects, and periodic re-evaluation of the patient is recommended to assess the overall benefit-to-risk ratio. Levodopa, pergolide, oxycodone, propoxyphene and carbamazepine were recommended as RLS treatments. Second-line recommended optional treatments include clonazepam, gabapentin, clonidine and iron. No specific recommendations were given for treatment of pregnant women or children with RLS, given the lack of adequate clinical data. Since this report more information has become available, particularly with respect to the new dopamine agonists pramipexole and ropinirole. These have the advantage of being relatively long lasting, having a good safety profile and being associated with what appears to be a reduced risk of augmentation.

On the available clinical evidence, most investigators consider the dopamine agonists pramipexole and ropinirole to be the first-line treatment for RLS symptoms severe enough to warrant pharmacologic treatment. Their effectiveness, side-effect profile and decreased risk of augmentation make them preferable to levodopa as initial therapy. They also avoid ergot-related side-effects found with the older dopamine agonists (bromocriptine, pergolide) such as pleural pulmonary fibrosis, retroperitoneal fibrosis and erythromelalgia. Other may choose carbergoline as initial therapy, given its long half-life and no reports of augmentation or rebound to date[79]. If dopamine agonists cannot be used or symptoms are infrequent, levodopa is a reasonable treatment as the risk of augmentation is lower with occasional dosing. Levodopa also provides rapid treatment benefits through its rapid onset of action (within 15 to 20 minutes of ingestion), whereas dopamine agonists typically require longer to reach peak effectiveness. Thus levodopa may be useful in patients with occasional symptoms that can be treated on an as-needed basis. Second-line therapies for patients who are not adequately controlled with a dopamine agonist or levodopa might include the anti-epileptic medications such as carbamazepine or gabapentin. These medications may be particularly suited for the treatment of RLS that is associated with a painful sensory component. Although benzodiazepines and opiates are also effective in treatment of RLS, their side-effect profile and risk of addiction limit their use. Benzodiazepines can be considered as alternatives to dopaminergic agents in the treatment of RLS associated with insomnia. In patients with moderate to severe RLS, there may be a need for combination therapies with two or more medications required in order to adequately control symptoms.

Figure 7.1 is a treatment algorithm for the management of RLS (based on the above). There are several limitations in the development of a treatment algorithm for RLS. There is a lack of large-scale, double-blind, long-term studies comparing the efficacy and long-term side-effects of the various agents and classes of medications used to treat RLS. It is difficult to

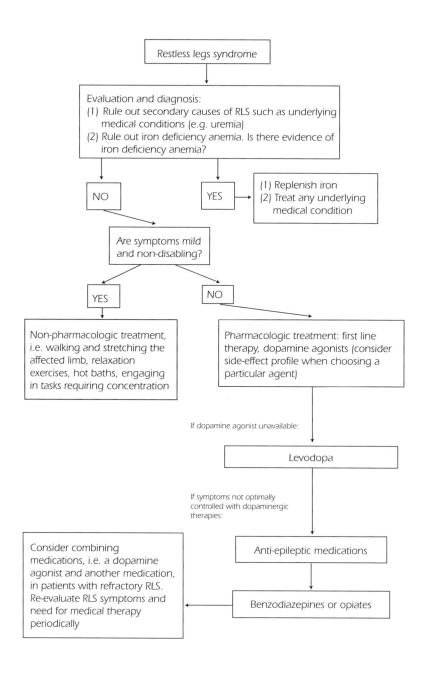

Figure 7.1 Treatment algorithm for restless legs syndrome

compare the different placebo-controlled trials that have been done to date, given the subjective nature of RLS symptoms and the lack (until recently) of standardized validated rating scales. Further, some studies have focused on subjective improvement in RLS symptoms whereas others have focused on improvement in objective polysomnographic measures such as PLMS number. Hence, comparative studies among and within the different classes of RLS medications have been very limited, and no studies comparing the newer dopamine agonists exist. Further studies will need to be done to assess the impact of RLS treatment on quality of life measures such as sleep disturbances, as well as to evaluate appropriate treatment for special populations such as pregnant women and children.

CONCLUSIONS

RLS is a common disorder that can occur as a primary disorder or in association with a number of other neurologic or metabolic disorders and can represent a source of disability to many patients. It remains unclear precisely how many patients have RLS, and how many have symptomatic forms that require pharmacologic treatment. Numerous agents have been shown to benefit RLS symptoms (see Table 7.1). Among these, dopaminergic agents are considered to be the most effective and accordingly to be the treatment of choice for RLS patients with sufficient severity of symptoms to warrant pharmacologic intervention. Dopamine agonists are generally the preferred initial treatment because of their long duration of action and reduced risk of the augmentation and rebound phenomena that complicate levodopa therapy. Antiepileptic medications such as gabapentin may have a role in the treatment of RLS, particularly in cases that fail dopaminergic treatment or have a severe pain component. Opioids and benzodiazepines are useful for the treatment of RLS but are limited by their side-effect profile. Controlled trials comparing the long-term safety and efficacy of the different dopamine agonists and other agents that are presently used in treating RLS still need to be done and may further shape our thinking on the management of this disorder. The role of various treatment combinations in patients with refractory RLS also needs to be further clarified. A flow chart providing a treatment algorithm for managing RLS is provided in Figure 7.1.

REFERENCES

1.   Willis T. *De Animae Brutorum*. London: Wells & Scott, 1672:339

2. Willis, T. *Two Discourses Concerning the Soul of Brutes*. London: Dring, Harper and Leigh, 1683

3. Ekbom KA. Restless legs: a clinical study. *Acta Med Scand* 1945;158 (Suppl):1–122

4. Lugaresi E, Coccagne G, Tassinari CA, Ambrosetto C. Polygraphic data on motor phenomena in the restless legs syndrome. *Rivisita Di Neurologia* 1965;35:550–61

5. Lugaresi E, Coccagna G, Gambi D, *et al*. A propos de quelques manifestations nocturnes myocloniques (nocturnal myoclonus de Symonds). *Rev Neurol* 1966;115:547

6. Montplaisir J, Godbout R. Nocturnal sleep of narcoleptic patients: revisited. *Sleep* 1986, 9:159–61

7. Schenck CH, Mahowald MW. Motor dyscontrol in narcolepsy: rapid-eye-movement sleep without atonia and REM sleep benhavior disorder. *Ann Neurol* 1992;32:3–10

8. Guilleminault C, *et al*. Periodic leg movement, sleep fragmentation and central sleep apnea in two cases: reduction with clonazepam. *Eur Respir J* 1988;1:762–5

9. Askenasy JJM. Sleep in Parkinson's disease. *Acta Neurol Scand* 1993;87:167–70

10. Phillips B, Young T, Finn L, *et al*. Epidemiology of restless legs symptoms in adults. *Arch Intern Med* 2000;160:2137–41

11. Lavigne GJ, Montplaisir JY. Restless legs syndrome and sleep bruxism: prevalence and association among Canadians. *Sleep* 1994;17:739–43

12. Chokroverty S, Jankovic J. Restless legs syndrome: a disease in search of identity. *Neurology* 1999;52:907–10

13. Ulfberg J, Nystrom B, Carter N, Edling C. Prevalence of restless legs syndrome among men aged 18–64 years: an association with somatic disease and neuropsychiatric symptoms. *Mov Disord* 2001;16:1159–63

14. Rotdach A, Trenkwalder C, Haberstock J, *et al*. Prevalence and risk factors of restless legs syndrome in an elderly population: the MEMO study. *Neurology* 2000;54:1064–8

15. Walters AS, Picchietti DL, Ehrenberg BL, Wagner ML. Restless legs syndrome in childhood and adolescence. *Pediatr Neurol* 1994;11:241–5

16. Walters AS, Hickey K, Maltzman J, *et al*. A questionnaire study of 138 patients with restless legs syndrome: the 'nightwalkers' survey. *Neurology* 1996;46:92–5

17. Montplaisir J, Boucher S, Poirier G, *et al*. Clinical, polysomnographic, and genetic characteristics of restless legs syndrome: a study of 133 patients diagnosed with new standard criteria. *Mov Disord* 1997;12:61–5

18. Winkelmann J, Wetter TC, Collado-Seidel V, *et al*. Frequency and characteristics of the hereditary restless legs syndrome in a population of 300 patients. *Sleep* 2000;23:597–602

19. Gemignani F, Marbini A. Restless legs syndrome and polyneuropathy (Comment). *J Neurol Neurosurg Psychiatry* 2002;72:555

20. Spillane JD, Nathan RW, Kelley RE, *et al.* Painful legs and moving toes. *Brain* 1971;94:541–56

21. Dressler D, Thompson PD, Gladhill RF, Marsden CD. The syndrome of painful legs and moving toes. *Mov Disord* 1994;9:13–21

22. Montagne P, Cirignotta F, Sacquegna T, *et al.* 'Painful legs and moving toes' associated with polyneuropathy. *J Neurol Neurosurg Psychiatry* 1983;46:399–403

23. Burke RE, Kang UJ, Jankovic J, *et al.* Tardive akathisia: an analysis of clinical features and response to open therapeutic trials. *Mov Disord* 1989;4:157–75

24. Lipinski JF, Hudson JI, Cunningham SL, *et al.* Polysomnographic characteristics of neuroleptic-induced akathisia. *Clin Neuropharmacol* 1991;14:413–19

25. Walters AS, Hening WA, Rubinstein M, *et al.* A clinical and polysomnographic comparison of neuroleptic-induced akathisia and idiopathic RLS. *Sleep* 1991;14:339–45

26. Lang AE, Johnson K. Akathisia in idiopathic Parkinson's disease. *Neurology* 1987;37:477–81

27. Connolly PS, *et al.* Treatment of nocturnal leg cramps: a crossover trial of quinine versus vitamin E. *Arch Intern Med* 1992;152:1877–80

28. Jacobsen JH, Rosenberg RS, Huttenlocher PR, *et al.* Familial nocturnal cramping. *Sleep* 1986;54–60

29. Weiner IH, Weiner HL. Nocturnal leg muscle cramps. *JAMA* 1980;244:2332–3

30. Dagnino N, *et al.* Hypnic physiologic myoclonus in man: an EEG-EMG study in normals and neurological patients. *Eur Neurol* 1985;2:47–58

31. Broughton R, Tolentino MA, Krelina M. Excessive fragmentary myoclonus in NREM sleep: a report of 38 cases. *Electroencephal Clin Neurophysiol* 1985;61:123–33

32. Chokroverty S, Walters AS, Zimmerman T, *et al.* Propiospinal myoclonus: a neurophysiological analysis. *Neurology* 1992;42:1591–5

33. Hopkins AP, Michael WF. Spinal myoclonus. *J Neurol Neurosurg Psychiatry* 1974;37:1112–15

34. Dhaliwal GS, McGreal DA. Spinal myoclonus in association with herpes zoster infection: two case reports. *Can J Neurol Sci* 1974;1:239–41

35. Hudson AJ, Brown WF, Gilbert JJ. Muscular pain-fasciculation syndrome. *Neurology* 1978;28:1105–9

36. Hudson AJ, Brown WF, Gilbert JJ. Muscular pain-fasciculation syndrome and restless legs [Letter]. *Neurology* 1979;29:907–8

37. Chesire WP. Hypotensive akathisia: autonomic failure associated with leg fidgeting while sitting. *Neurology* 2000;55:1923–6

38. Bhatia KP, Bhatt MH, Marsden CD. The causalgia-dystonia syndrome. *Brain* 1993;116:843–51

39. Schenck CH. Restless legs syndrome and periodic leg movements of sleep: global therapeutic considerations. *Sleep Med Rev* 2002;6:247–51

40. Kales A, Soldatos CR, Kales JD. Taking a sleep history. *Am Fam Physician* 1980;22:101–8

41. Berkowitz HL. Restless legs syndrome disguised as an affective disorder. *Psychosomatics* 1984;25:336–7

42. Ekbom KA. Restless legs: a clinical study. *Acta Med Scand Suppl* 1995;158:1

43. Clark M. Restless legs syndrome. *J Am Board Fam Pract* 2001;14:368–74

44. Allen RP, Walters AS. Restless legs syndrome diagnosis and management. In Chokroverty S, Hening WA, Walters AS, eds. *Sleep and Movement Disorders.* Philadelphia: Butterworth Heinemann, 2003:341–7

45. Chesson AL, Wise M, Davila D, *et al.* Practice parameters for the treatment of restless legs syndrome and periodic limb movement disorder. *Sleep* 1999;22:961–8

46. Rye DB, Delong MR. Amelioration of sensory limb discomfort of restless legs syndrome by pallidotomy. *Ann Neurol* 1999;46:800–1

47. Akpinar S. Restless legs treatment with dopaminergic drugs. *Clin Neuropharmacol* 1987;10:69–79

48. Brodeur C, Montplaisir J, Godbout R, Marinier R. Treatment of restless legs syndrome and periodic movements during sleep with L-dopa: a double-blind, controlled study. *Neurology* 1988;38:1845–8

49. Hening W, Allen R, Earley C, *et al.* The treatment of restless legs syndrome and periodic limb movement disorder. *Sleep* 1999;22:970–99

50. Trenkwalder C, Stiasny K, Pollmacher T, *et al.* L-dopa therapy of uremic and idiopathic restless legs syndrome: a double-blind, crossover trial. *Sleep* 1995;18:681–8

51. Benes H, Kurella B, Kummer B, *et al.* Rapid onset of action of levodopa in a restless legs syndrome: a double-blind, randomized, multicenter, crossover trial. *Sleep* 1999;22:1073–81

52. von Scheele C, Kempi V. Long-term effect of dopaminergic drugs in restless legs syndrome. A two year follow-up. *Arch Neurol* 1990;47:1223–4

53. Guilleminault C, Cetel M, Philip P. Dopaminergic treatment of restless legs and rebound phenomenom. *Neurology* 1993;43:445

54. Becker PM, Jamieson AO, Brown WD. Dopaminergic agents in restless legs syndrome and periodic limb movements of sleep: response and complications of extended treatment in 49 cases. *Sleep* 1993;16:713–16

55. Collado-Seidel V, Kazenwadel J, Wetter TC, *et al.* A controlled study of additional sr-L-dopa in L-dopa responsive RLS with late night symptoms. *Neurology* 1999;52:225–90

56. Allen RP, Earley CJ. Augmentation of the restless legs syndrome with carbidopa/levodopa. *Sleep* 1996;19:205–13

57. Silber MH, Shepard JW Jr, Wisbey JA. Pergolide in the management of restless legs syndrome: an extended study. *Sleep* 1997;20:878–82

58. Staedt J, Hunerjager H, Ruther E, Stoppe G. Pergolide: treatment of choice in restless legs syndrome (RLS) and nocturnal myoclonus syndrome (NMS): long-term follow-up on pergolide. *J Neural Transm* 1998;105:265–8

59. Earley CJ. Restless legs syndrome. *N Engl J Med* 2003;348:2103–9

60. Walters AS, Hening WA, Kavey N, *et al*. A double-blind randomized crossover trial of bromocriptine and placebo in RLS. *Ann Neurol* 1988;24:455–8

61. Odin P, Mrowka M, Shing M. Restless legs syndrome. *Eur J Neurol* 2002;9(Suppl 3):59–67

62. Wetter TC, Stiasny K, Winkelmann J, *et al*. A randomized controlled study of pergolide in patients with restless legs syndrome. *Neurology* 1999;52:944–50

63. Earley CJ, Allen RP. Pergolide and carbidopa/levodopa treatment of the restless legs syndrome and periodic leg movements in sleep in a consecutive series of patients. *Sleep* 1996;19:801–10

64. Earley W, Yaffee JB, Allen RP. Randomized, double-blind, placebo-controlled trial of pergolide in restless legs syndrome. *Neurology* 1998;51:1599–602

65. Staedt J, Wassmuth F, Ziemann U, *et al*. Pergolide: treatment of choice in restless legs syndrome (RLS) and nocturnal myoclonus syndrome (NMS). A double-blind randomized crossover trial of pergolide versus levodopa. *J Neural Trans* 1997:104:461–8

66. Montplasir J, Nicolas A, Denesle R, *et al*. Restless legs syndrome improved by pramipexole: a double-blind randomized trial. *Neurology* 1999;52:938–43

67. Montplaisir J, Denesle R, Petit D. Pramipexole in the treatment of restless legs syndrome: a follow-up study. *Eur J Neurol* 2000;7:27–31

68. Lin SC, Kaplan J, Burger CD, Fredrickson PA. Effect of pramipexole treatment of resistant restless legs syndrome. *Mayo Clinic Proc* 1998;73:497–500

69. Ferini-Strambi L, Oldani A, Castronovo V, Zucconi M. RLS augmentation and pramipexole long-term treatment. *Neurology* 2001;56 (Suppl 3):A20 (Abstract)

70. Comella CL. Restless legs syndrome: treatment with dopaminergic agents. *Neurology* 2002;58 (Suppl 1):S87–92

71. Silber MH, Girish M, Izurieta R. Pramipexole in the management of restless legs syndrome: an extended study. *Sleep* 2001;24:A18

72. Winkelman JW, Johnston L. Augmentation and tolerance with long-term pramipexole treatment of restless legs syndrome (RLS). *Sleep Med* 2004;5:9–14

73. Ondo W. Ropinirole for restless legs syndrome. *Mov Disord* 1999;14:138–40

74. Saletu B, Gruber G, Saletu M, *et al*. Sleep laboratory studies in restless legs syndrome as compared with normals and acute effects of ropinirole. 1. Findings on objective and subjective sleep and awakening quality. *Neuropsychobiology* 2000;41:181–9

75. Trenkwalder C, Garcia-Borreguero D, Montagna P, *et al*. Ropinirole in the treatment of restless legs syndrome: results from the TREAT RLS 1 study, a 12 week, randomized, placebo controlled study in 10 European countries. *J Neurol Neurosurg Psychiatry* 2004;75:92–7

76. Stiasny K, Robbecke J, Schuler P, Oertel WH. Treatment of idiopathic restless legs syndrome (RLS) with the D2 agonist cabergoline – an open-label clinical trial. *Sleep* 2000;23:349–54

77. Stiasny K, Ueberal MA, Oertel WH. Cabergoline in RLS: a double-blind placebo-controlled multi-center dose finding trial. *Sleep* 2000;25(Suppl):A489

78. Stegie F, Metcalf P, Dhawan V, *et al*. The side-effect profile of cabergoline, an ergot agonist; a clinical follow-up study in Parkinson's disease and restless legs syndrome. *Mov Disord* 2004;in press

79. Chaudhuri KR. Restless legs syndrome. *N Engl J Med* 2003;349:815

80. Stiasny K, Benes H, Bodenschatz R, *et al*., the RTG Study Group. Rotigotine CDS (Constant Delivery System) in the treatment of moderate to advanced stages of restless legs syndrome: a double-blind, placebo-controlled pilot study. *Mov Disord* 2002;17 (Suppl 5):S241

81. Reuter I, Ellis CM, Chaudhuri KR. Nocturnal subcutaneous apomorphine infusion in Parkinson's disease and restless legs syndrome. *Acta Neurol Scand* 1999;100:163–7

82. Peled R, Lavie P. Double-blind evaluation of clonazepam on periodic leg movements in sleep. *J Neurol Neurosurg Psychiatry* 1987;50:1679–81

83. Telstad W, Sorenson O, Larsen S, *et al*. Treatment of the restless legs syndrome with carbamazepine: a double-blind study. *BMJ* 1984;288:444–6

84. Zucconi M, Coccagna G, Petronelli R *et al*. Nocturnal myoclonus in restless legs syndrome effect of carbamazepine treatment. *Funct Neurol* 1989;4:263–71

85. Garcia-Borreguero D, Larrosa O, de la Llave Y, *et al*. Treatment of the restless legs syndrome with gabapentin: a double-blind, cross-over study. *Neurology* 2002;59:1573–9

86. Happe S, Sauter C, Klosch G, *et al*. Gapapentin versus ropinirole in the treatment of idiopathic restless legs syndrome. *Neuropsychobiology* 2003;48:82–6

87. Ehrenberg BL, Eisensehr I, Corbett KE, *et al*. Valproate for sleep consolidation in periodic limb movement disorder. *J Clin Psychopharmacol* 2000;20:574–8

88. Walters AS, Wagner ML, Hening WA, *et al*. Successful treatment of the idiopathic RLS in a randomized double-blind trial of oxycodone versus placebo. *Sleep* 1993;16:327–32

89. Allen RP, Kaplan PW, Buchholz DW, *et al*. Double-blinded, placebo-controlled comparison of high dose propoxyphene and moderate dose carbidopa/levodopa for the treatment of periodic limb movements in sleep. *Sleep Res* 1992;21:166

90. Kaplan P, Allen R, Buchholz D, Walters J. A double-blind, placebo-controlled study of the treatment of periodic limb movements using carbidopa/levodopa and propoxyphene. *Sleep* 1993;16:717–23

91. Hening WA, Walters AS. Successful long-term therapy of the RLS with opioid medications [Abstract]. *Sleep Res* 1989;18:241

92. Earley CJ, Connor JR, Beard JL, *et al*. Abnormalities in CSF concentrations of ferritin and transferrin in restless legs syndrome. *Neurology* 2000;54: 1698–7000

93. O' Keefe ST, Gavin K, Lavan JN. Iron status and restless legs syndrome in the elderly. *Age Ageing* 1994;23:200–3

94. Allen RP, Earley CJ. Dopamine and iron in the restless legs syndrome. In Chokroverty S, Hening WA,Walters AS, eds. *Sleep and Movement Disorders*. Philadelphia: Butterworth Heinemann, 2003:333–40

95. Davis BJ, Rajput A, Rajput ML, *et al*. A randomized, double-blind placebo-controlled trial of iron in restless legs syndrome. *Eur Neurol* 2000;43:70–5

96. Nordlander NB. Restless legs. *Br J Phys Med* 1954;17:160–2

97. Wagner M, Walters AS, Coleman RG, *et al*. Randomized, double-blind study of clonidine in restless legs syndrome. *Sleep* 1996;19:52–8

98. Guilleminault C, Flagg W. Effect of baclofen on sleep-related periodic leg movements. *Ann Neurol* 1984;15:234–9

99. Sharif AA. Entacapone in restless legs syndrome. *Mov Disord* 2002;17:421

8   Augmentation and rebound

K. Ray Chaudhuri

AUGMENTATION

In RLS, initially there is often a dramatic response to treatment with dopamine agonists or levodopa. However, this beneficial response may not be sustained. One complication, thought to arise from dopaminergic drug administration, appears to be augmentation, first recognized by Allen and Early in 1996[1]. They reported that 82% of their patients treated with a night-time dose of levodopa/carbidopa over a period of 2 months reported that RLS symptoms had increased in late afternoon and early evening. The symptoms were severe in some cases and required a change in medication. In general, it is now recognized that augmentation complicates about 80% of patients with RLS on chronic levodopa treatment. Clinically, augmentation may start about 3–4 weeks after starting treatment and this is accompanied by an increase in symptom severity or a decrease in drug efficacy. Increasing doses of levodopa may lead to increasing augmentation, and discontinuation of treatment unmasks the symptoms of RLS. However, augmentation usually resolves on withdrawal of the drug.

Clinically, augmentation presents with symptoms of RLS which:
(1) are of increased severity;
(2) are more easily provoked;
(3) occur earlier in the day or in the afternoon; and
(4) spread to upper limbs.

Increasing the dose of the drug which causes augmentation often worsens symptoms and may result in the patient suffering from RLS symptoms day and night. Pain may be an associated feature and sleeplessness may produce a severe anxiety state. The symptoms may cause acute inner restlessness and may resemble the syndrome of akathisia commonly seen with neuroleptic drugs. The trunk may be affected and involvement of upper limbs and trunk may mimic a spinal cord syndrome. The causation is poorly understood and its relationship to levodopa is somewhat similar to dyskinesias which develop in Parkinson's disease after exposure to levodopa. Risk factors appear to be early pre-treatment in the evening and doses of levodopa beyond 200 mg.

Augmentation appears not to be exclusive to levodopa. Early and Allen[2] and Silber *et al.*[3] also described augmentation with the use of the dopamine agonist pergolide in 15–25% of cases. More recently, Ferini-Strambi[4] has described augmentation in 8.3% of cases of RLS treated with the non-ergot dopamine agonist pramipexole. Augmentation was commoner in secondary RLS and occurred 4–15 weeks after treatment. However, in another clinical follow-up study, Montplaisir and colleagues[5] noted that there was no augmentation with pramipexole at 7.8 months follow-up in seven RLS patients. The jury is, therefore, still out in relation to augmentation and pramipexole. Currently, there are no reports of augmentation with the use of cabergoline or ropinirole. The key features of augmentation are also referred to in Chapter 2.

REBOUND

The rebound phenomenon was originally identified by Guilleminault *et al.*[6] and describes the reappearance of RLS symptoms after the drug dose has worn off. It is in many ways similar to the 'end-of-dose' or 'wearing-off' phenomenon seen in Parkinson's disease. Clinically, this manifests as RLS symptoms occurring in early morning or late at night after the night-time/evening drug dose is no longer effective.

DIAGNOSIS

Diagnosis of rebound and augmentation is important, as non-recognition will lead to ineffective treatment. Both symptoms are diagnosed clinically, and asking the patient to keep a symptom diary may be particularly useful. These complications usually occur 3–4 months after initiation of treatment. Rebound may lead to very poor sleep, and upper limb or trunk symptoms with augmentation may be misdiagnosed as psychiatric symptoms or akathisia. Recently, Garcia-Borreguero and colleagues (Chapter 9)[7] have been developing a specific augmentation severity rating scale which is currently in the process of being validated.

TREATMENT

Augmentation is usually seen with levodopa used at doses above 200 mg/day. Severe augmentation requires discontinuation of levodopa whereas mild symptoms may be treated by reduction of dose. Increasing doses of levodopa will worsen augmentation. However, as a general rule, once augmentation appears it is best to use an alternative agent, perhaps a dopamine agonist, or to switch from one dopamine agonist to another. Some clinicians have tried alternate dosing with levodopa and dopamine agonists. In intermittent RLS, an 'as and when necessary' dosing regime of levodopa or dopamine agonists may avoid augmentation.

Rebound appears to be related to the half-life of the drug used, the short half-life of levodopa causing symptoms in early morning. In our clinical practice, cabergoline appears to be the best drug to counteract rebound as it has the longest half-life and, given at night-time, successfully controls symptoms during the night and day[7]. An alternative strategy may be to use shorter half-life agonists three times a day.

REFERENCES

1. Allen RP, Earley CJ. Augmentation of the restless legs syndrome with car-bidopa/levodopa. *Sleep* 1996;19:205–13

2. Earley CJ, Allen RP. Pergolide and carbidopa/levodopa treatment of the rest-less legs syndrome and periodic leg movements in sleep in a consecutive series of patients. *Sleep* 1996;19:801–10

3. Silber MH, Shepard Jr JW, Wisbey JA. Pergolide in the management of restless legs syndrome: an extended study. *Sleep* 1997;20:878–82

4. Ferini-Strambi L. Restless legs syndrome augmentation and pramipexole treat-ment. *Sleep Med* 2002;3:S23–25

5. Montplaisir J, Denesle R, Petit D. Pramipexole in the treatment of restless legs syndrome: a follow up study. *Eur J Neurol* 2000;7(Suppl 1):27–31

6. Guilleminault C, Cetel M, Philip P. Dopaminergic treatment of restless legs and rebound phenomenon. *Neurology* 1993;43:445

7. Chaudhuri KR. The restless legs syndrome: time to recognize a very common movement disorder. *Pract Neurol* 2003;3:204–13

9 Diagnosis of the restless legs syndrome: the use of the sleep laboratory

D. Garcia-Borreguero, C. Serrano and R. Egatz

INTRODUCTION

Because of the subjective nature of the clinical features of restless legs syndrome (RLS), the diagnosis of RLS is usually based on the patient's clinical history[1]. Thus, a recent international workshop on the diagnosis and epidemiology of RLS, sponsored by the National Institutes of Health, defined four essential diagnostic criteria, all of which can be assessed by clinical history alone[2]. These criteria are:

(1) A compelling urge to move the limbs, usually (although not necessarily) associated with paresthesias and dysesthesias. The discomfort is often described in terms such as: creeping, crawling, itching, burning, searing, tugging, pulling, drawing, aching, heat/coldness, 'electric current like', restlessness or pain, and seems to be located deep in the muscle or bone, and more seldom in joints[3]. The sensory symptoms involve the legs, but in almost half of the patients the arms also. The discomfort can occur unilaterally or bilaterally.

(2) The urge to move and the unpleasant sensations are exclusively present, or at least most severe, at rest or inactivity. Once the patient is lying or sitting, the symptoms begin with a delay of some minutes to 1 hour[4]. Typical situations where the symptoms are present include, apart from lying in bed or sitting in a chair, the passive rest of longer journeys in a car or plane, as well as visits to the theater and cinema. In advanced cases such activities are almost impossible. The symptoms often become more intense after longer periods of rest.

(3) The urge to move or the unpleasant sensations are partially or totally relieved by movement, at least as long as the activity continues. In milder cases the patient might not have to get up to walk; it might be sufficient to move in the bed or chair.

(4) A circadian rhythm with worsening of the urge to move or of the unpleasant symptoms during the evening and/or night can be established. In a typical case, the untreated patient reaches maximal severity of symptoms between 11 p.m. and 4 a.m. and maximal relief between

6 and 12 a.m. The night-time worsening occurs whether the patient is asleep or not.

Apart from these essential diagnostic criteria, the NIH criteria include three supportive, but not obligatory, clinical features: (1) a positive response to dopaminergic medication; (2) periodic limb movements during sleep (PLMS), PLMS occur in over 80% of the patients[5,6]; and (3) a family history of RLS.

More than 90% of patients report difficulties in initiating or maintaining sleep[7]. In sleep laboratory investigations it has been possible to verify increased sleep latency and PLMS-associated arousals/awakenings, together with a decrease in total sleep time, sleep efficiency and slow-wave sleep. Patients frequently sleep less than 50% of the time spent in bed.

When typical symptoms are present, the diagnosis is easy to make. However, it can be more difficult in patients with either atypical symptomatology or co-morbidity with other sleep or movement disorders. In such cases, sleep laboratory tests can be of help. The diagnosis is further supported if there is a response to dopaminergic medication.

In this chapter, we review the diagnostic value of sleep laboratory tests for RLS.

POLYSOMNOGRAPHY (SLEEP STUDIES)

As well as symptoms during the waking time, the vast majority of patients with RLS have stereotyped repetitive movements when they are asleep. These movements are known as periodic limb movements during sleep (PLMS). Since they occur while the patient is asleep, their presence can only be confirmed during sleep studies (Figure 9.1).

PLMS are rhythmical extensions of the big toe and dorsiflexions of the ankle, with occasional flexions of the knee and hip. Each movement lasts approximately 0.5–5 s with a frequency of one every 20–40 s. PLMS appear in clusters of at least four movements, with an inter-movement interval between 5 and 90 s. PLMS are in general more frequent during the first half of the night, as they are more common during sleep stages 1 and 2 (Figure 9.2). However, PLMS can be present during the entire sleep period.

When PLMS are intense, they can cause electroencephalogram (EEG) arousals (Figure 9.3). If these PLM arousals are numerous, PLMS alone can lead to non-restorative sleep. When evaluating sleep studies, the PLM-index (PLMI) is defined as the number of PLMS per hour of sleep. It is a matter

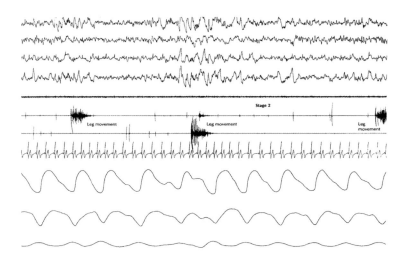

Figure 9.1   Periodic sequence of leg movements during sleep

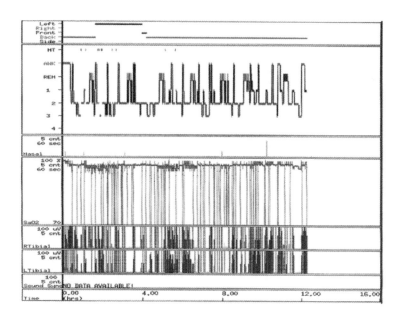

Figure 9.2   Sleep fragmentation due to periodic limb movements during sleep

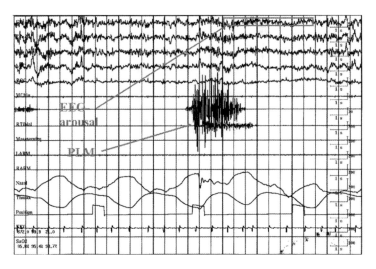

Figure 9.3   Electroencephalogram (EEC) arousal due to periodic limb movements (PLM) during sleep

of discussion which PLMI is abnormal, but a recent study has established the threshold at 11/hour[8].

However, the presence of a high number of PLMS is by no means specific to RLS, as PLMS co-occur in a wide range of sleep/wake complaints, including narcolepsy, sleep apnea and REM sleep behavior disorder. Other authors have found PLMS in otherwise physically and mentally healthy subjects. PLMS can also occur during sleep but without any sensory-motor symptoms while awake. The disorder is then called periodic limb movement disorder (PLMD), and should not be confounded with PLMS in RLS, as both disorders might represent separate nosological entities.

Furthermore, as many as 12% of RLS patients do not have marked PLMS when recorded for two or more nights[5]. When recording for two consecutive nights, a PLMI cut-off score of 11/hour provides a diagnostic sensitivity and specificity of approximately 80%[9]. Thus, the presence of an abnormal number of PLMS during a polysomnography supports a clinical diagnosis, but does not suffice by itself to establish a firm diagnosis.

PLMI can be used to assess disease severity, although sleep efficiency, another parameter obtained routinely during PSG, has been shown to correlate better with clinical ratings of RLS[10]. Sleep efficiency is defined as the percentage of total sleep time out of total recording time. However, although sleep efficiency might reflect RLS severity, it is considered to be a very unspecific marker of disturbed sleep.

Methods in polysomnography

Polysomnography (PSG) is defined as the recording of multiple physiologic variables during sleep[11,12]. This diagnostic technique is an important tool in the evaluation of patients with sleep-related movement disorders, especially when the medical history is insufficient to provide a definitive diagnosis. PSG allows periodic limb movements (PLM) to be identified and quantified. Furthermore, if an extended electroencephalographic coverage (i.e. 12 or more channels) of the scalp is used and a videotape recording (video-EEG) is performed, PSG can be helpful in identifying an epileptic origin of sleep-related movement disorders. Respiratory events and cardiac function can be recorded using specific montages, that include airflow parameters and ECG[11,12].

When used for monitoring of sleep-related movement disorders, PSG consists of a simultaneous recording of EEG, electro-oculogram (EOG) and surface electromyogram (EMG) under synchronized video-recording during sleep. In most cases, in order to exclude sleep-related breathing disturbance, additional physiologic variables such as electrocardiogram, respiratory flow and effort, and continuous oxyhemoglobin saturation are recorded simultaneously (Figures 9.1–9.3). However, PSG can in principle include any physiologic variable that can be recorded and amplified through AC/DC amplifiers.

Electroencephalogram

The EEG measures the difference in electrical potential between pairs of electrodes placed on the scalp. These signals, reflecting synchronous post-synaptic potentials in large groups of neurons, are amplified and filtered to produce an analog or digital recording.

The EEG electrodes for overnight studies are generally attached to the scalp using small patches of gauze soaked in collodium and dried with compressed air. The conducting medium may be added through a small hole in the electrode cup before application, and an airtight seal will prevent evaporation for at least 24–36 h (Figure 9.4). C3 and C4 leads are conventionally used to record EEG, and these are referenced to a neutral electrode on the contralateral mastoid or ear lobe (Figure 9.5). In addition, some laboratories routinely record occipital (O1/A2 or O2/A1) and frontal EEG channels. Sleep stage scoring does not usually require measurement of focal EEG activity or regional comparisons.

Electro-oculogram

Eye movements are recorded to determine REM stage (phasic bursts of rapid eye movements), as well as slow eye movements during the onset of

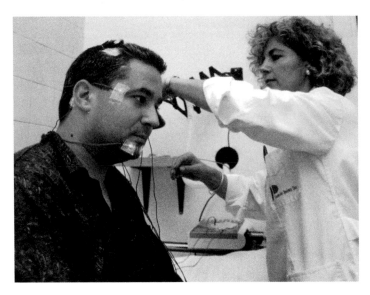

Figure 9.4 Preparation of a patient for a sleep study

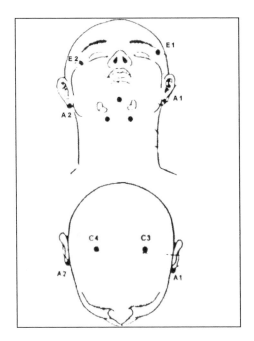

Figure 9.5 Placement of electroencephalogram, electro-oculogram and submental electro-myogram electrodes for sleep recording

sleep. The EOG recordings are based on a small electropotential difference from the front to the back of the eye. Standard EOG placements include the right outer canthus (ROC), and the left outer canthus (LOC) (Figure 9.5).

Submental electromyogram
The EMG from muscles beneath the chin is used as a criterion for staging REM sleep (Figure 9.5).

Anterior tibialis muscle EMG
Limb EMG recordings are especially important in RLS and PLMD. For leg-movement recordings, electrodes are placed over the anterior tibialis muscle, approximately 2–4 cm apart (Figure 9.6). Because movements may occur only in one leg or alternate between the two legs throughout the night, activity in both legs should be recorded. Calibration should be performed before recording by having patients slowly dorsiflex and plantarflex the great toe of each foot to approximately 30 degrees.

When the study is scored, sleep stages are described as follows:

Relaxed wakefulness Eyes closed: rhythmic alpha (8–13 Hz), prominent in occipital, attenuates with attention. Eyes open: relatively low voltage, mixed frequency (Figure 9.7).

Non-REM-sleep

Stage 1   Relatively low voltage, mixed frequency. Can be theta (3–7 Hz) activity with greater amplitude. Vertex sharp waves. Syncronous high-voltage theta bursts in children (Figure 9.8).

Stage 2   Background with relatively low voltage, and mixed frequency. Sleep spindles (12–14 Hz). K complex (≥ 0.5 s) (Figure 9.9).

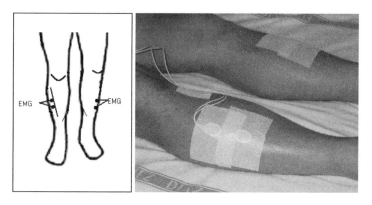

Figure 9.6   Placement of m. anterior tibialis leads

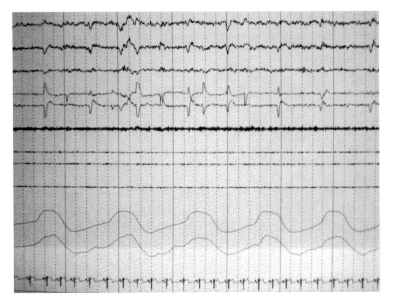

Figure 9.7 Relaxed wakefulness

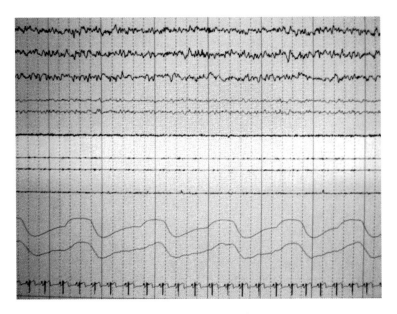

Figure 9.8 Non-rapid eye movement sleep stage 1

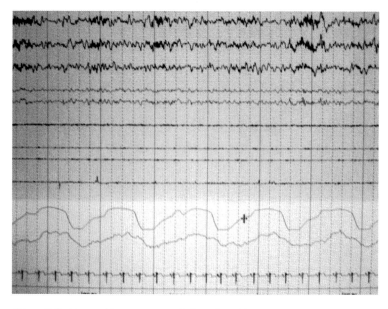

Figure 9.9 Non-rapid eye movement sleep stage 2

Stage 3   High amplitude waves (> 75 μV), slow frequency, in 20–50% of the 30-s epoch (Figure 9.10).

Stage 4   High amplitude waves (> 75 μV), slow frequency, in > 50% of the epoch.

REM-sleep Relatively low voltage, mixed frequency EEG in conjunction with episodic REMs and low amplitude of the EMG (Figure 9.11).

Movement time (MT) This is defined as a period in which the record is obscured by the movement of the subject, and the epochs scored precede or follow sleep stages. EEG and EOG tracings are obscured in more than half the epoch by muscle tension and/or amplifier blocking artifacts associated with movements of the subject.

In summary, even though RLS is diagnosed by means of clinical criteria, PSG remains an important tool in the evaluation of RLS, and is used in most sleep laboratories around the world. Performing PSG is recommended in patients with probable or definite RLS in cases where[13]:

• Based on the patient's history and on clinical symptoms, RLS is probable, but symptoms may appear atypical or be affected by other disorders.

• There is an ongoing severe insomnia and/or a lack of efficacy in patients with typical RLS symptoms during treatment with sufficient dosages of dopaminergic drugs (dopamine agonists or 250 mg L-dopa).

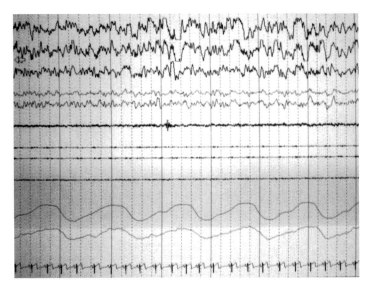

Figure 9.10   Non-rapid eye movement sleep stage 3

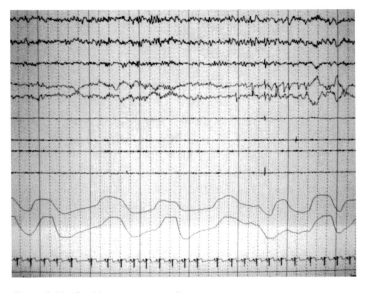

Figure 9.11   Rapid eye movement sleep

- The patient complains about daytime sleepiness as a leading symptom, in order to rule out other causes of daytime sleepiness.
- The patient is younger than 30 years of age, suffers from severe RLS and should be treated daily with dopaminergic substances, in order to support the diagnosis with the prospect of a life-long treatment with medication.
- The patient suffers from severe RLS and an opioid medication is conceivable. In this case, the severity of insomnia and the occurrence of PLMS should be documented, and a pre-existing sleep-related respiratory disorder that might worsen during treatment should be excluded.
- The patient is diagnosed as having RLS and an additional sleep-related disorder, but complains about persistence of symptoms of RLS during pharmacotherapy.
- An expert's report is needed for legal purposes.

PSG remains an important but costly method of assessment of RLS patients. However, because of its cost, it should be reserved for patients with specific diagnostic and therapeutic indications. Additional, less expensive, instrumental assessment tools have been developed over recent years and might offer promising alternatives for the future.

SUGGESTED IMMOBILIZATION TEST (SIT)

RLS symptoms are primarily observed during wakefulness, especially when the patient is at rest during the evening or at night. With this aspect in mind, objective tests have been tried to assess symptoms during wakefulness. Because sensitive symptoms are, owing to their subjective nature, difficult to assess, efforts have focused on the assessment of motor symptoms during wakefulness. Periodic leg movements also occur during wakefulness (PLMW) (Figure 9.12), particularly when patients are lying in bed attempting to remain quiet[14–16]. The periodicity of PLMW is similar to that of PLMS. However, during the change from wakefulness to stage 1 and stage 2 sleep, the inter-movement interval of the periodic leg movements gradually increases, and the duration of the movement decreases. In one study performed in 110 RLS subjects, the inter-movement interval during wakefulness was 16 s, against 19.6 s for stage 1, 26.4 s for stage 2, and 29.2 s for stages 3 and 4[15]. Simultaneously, variability of the inter-movement interval decreases from wakefulness to deeper sleep[9].

The occurrence of PLMW during waking and the quiescegenic nature of RLS provided the basis for developing a test aimed to be more specific to

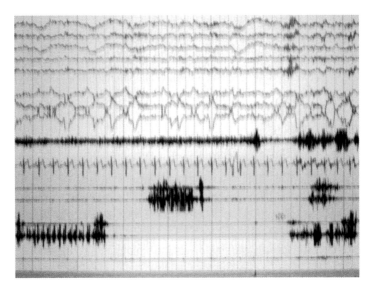

Figure 9.12 *Periodic limb movements during wakefulness*

RLS than PLMS in sleep studies. This test is the suggested immobilization test (SIT), and was developed by Montplaisir and colleagues to be used for diagnosis and evaluation of the severity of RLS[9]. The SIT is a 60-min test, to be performed in the evening 90 min before bedtime, during which patients recline in bed at a 45° angle with their eyes open and legs stretched out. Patients are instructed not to move or to fall asleep. Leg activity is recorded using standard bilateral anterior tibialis surface EMG (Figure 9.13). EEGs are simultaneously recorded to ensure that the patient remains awake. In addition, patients are asked, every 5 min for the entire hour, to fill in a visual analog scale for sensorial discomfort in their legs (Figure 9.14).

PLMW during SIT are scored according to the same criteria as those used for PLMS[17], but include a few modifications. Thus, any movements lasting between 0.5 and 10 s are scored, and the inter-movement interval is 4–90 s. PLM are scored as bilateral if the interval between the offset of movement in one leg and the onset of movement in the other leg is lower than 4 s. The use of these criteria differentiates PLMW from myoclonia (by their duration) and from continued EMG tonic bursts (by the required inter-movement intervals). Furthermore, according to Coleman's criteria, any leg movements to be scored have to be part of a series of at least four consecutive movements and thus be periodic. However, during wakefulness the longest duration for leg movement to be scored as such is 10 s, whereas

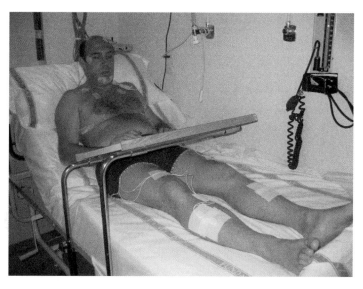

Figure 9.13 Suggested immobilization test (SIT)

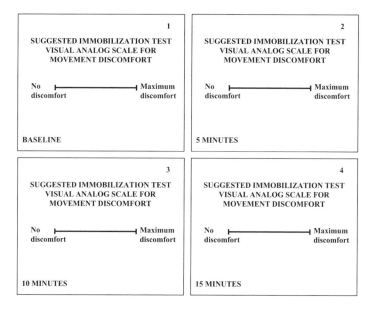

Figure 9.14 Visual analog scale for movement discomfort

during sleep the maximal duration is 5 s. The longer duration of leg movements during wakefulness is justified as being the result of a voluntary contraction of leg muscles that follows the shorter, involuntary contraction, in order to relieve the dysesthesias. Dysesthesias usually take place within 2 s of the onset of PLMW[18,19]. Thus, PLMW and dysesthesias should be considered as being part of the same motor rhythm.

PLMW are more common during the second half of the SIT both in patients and controls, but the difference was significant only in RLS patients ($p < 0.05$)[19], suggesting that PLM increased with increasing duration of immobility. Tables 9.1 and 9.2 summarize these modified criteria that are used to record and score PLMW during SIT.

As mentioned above, a visual analog scale on leg discomfort (Figure 9.14) is usually administered every 5 min during the SIT. Ideally, the visual analog scale is connected to an electronic device that provides an auditory signal every 5 min, at which time the patient has to estimate with a moving pointer his level of leg discomfort on a 100-mm horizontal bar. The descriptors 'no discomfort' and 'extreme discomfort' are used at the left and right endpoints of the visual analog scale. The device converts the rating automatically into a 0–100 scale. Thus, 12 values are obtained during each SIT. The mean leg discomfort score (SIT-MDS) represents the average value of

Table 9.1   Criteria for scoring periodic leg movement syndrome during polysomnography (adapted from Coleman et al., 1980)[17]

1.	Series of at least four or more consecutive leg movements
2.	Duration of leg movement between 0.5 and 5 s
3.	Duration of inter-movement interval (IMI) between 4 and 90 s

Table 9.2   Criteria for scoring periodic leg movements while awake (PLMW)[9] during the suggested immobilization test (SIT) (adapted from Coleman et al., 1980)[17]

1.	Series of at least four or more consecutive leg movements
2.	Duration of leg movement between 0.5 and 10 s
3.	Duration of inter-movement interval (IMI) between 4 and 90 s

these 12 measures. The maximum leg discomfort value (SIT D_{max}) corresponds to the highest value recorded during SIT.

A prospective study by the same group administered the SIT followed by a PSG to 19 RLS patients and 19 controls[19]. RLS patients had a significantly higher PLMS index on PSG (57.1 ± 40.1, $p < 0.00002$) than controls. On the SIT, PLMW index (88.4 ± 62.6, $p < 0.00002$), SIT-MDS (32.6 ± 15.1, $p < 0.00001$) and SIT D_{max} (63.4 ± 27.4, $p < 0.00001$) were also higher than controls but correlation analyses found no significant relationship between any of these measures. Both SIT-MDS and SIT-PLM indexes worsened significantly across time during the 60-min test ($p < 0.0001$ and $p < 0.00001$, respectively): 84% of RLS patients experienced their SIT D_{max} during the second half of the test. The existence of a voluntary and an involuntary component in movements could explain the discrepancy between a high value in SIT-MDS and a low value in SIT-PLM in some patients, as results depend considerably on the effort applied by patients to keep their legs immobile. Thus, at least partial aspects of leg movements are under voluntary control.

The SIT has been validated in a sample of severely affected patients and controls. Using a cut-off value of PLMW index > 40, it provides both a high sensitivity ($81 \pm 19\%$) and a high specificity ($81 \pm 19\%$) for the diagnosis of severe RLS. If the utility of SIT-MDS is confirmed by future studies, it could be used alone to support the clinical diagnosis of RLS and, since it is a simple and inexpensive method, it could even be used in the home environment.

In a later study, Michaud and co-workers[8] compared several PSG parameters (PLMS index, PLMW index and PLMS-arousal index) with SIT parameters (PLMW index and SIT-MDS) in 100 RLS patients and 50 controls. Applying a cut-off value of 11 in SIT-MDS, 12 in SIT-PLM index and 15 in PLMW index, a positive correlation between SIT-MDS and SIT-PLM index ($r = 0.33$; $p = 0.001$) was found. In addition, they reported a trend for significance between the SIT-PLM index and the PSG-PLMW index ($r = 0.25$; $p < 0.01$). The highest sensitivities were obtained with the PSG-PLMW index (87%), followed by SIT-MDS (82%). The study of the area under receiver–operation curves for each parameter revealed that the PLMW index on PSG discriminated best patients from controls (area under curve 91.7%), followed by SIT-MDS (88.3%). If PLMW index on PSG and SIT-MDS were used in combination, a sensitivity of 82% and a specificity of 100% were achieved (88% of subjects correctly classified). These parameters were followed by the PSG-PLMS index, the SIT-PLMW index and the PSG-PLMS-arousal index (correctly classified 77.3%, 69.9% and 68% of all subjects, respectively); all these parameters yielded a specificity over 80% except for the PSG-PLMS index, which was the least specific (76%).

It should be noted that these results are based on comparisons between RLS patients and normal controls. It is conceivable that a comparison with insomnia patients or other sleep or pain disorders would reduce the specificity and sensitivity even further. Thus, as mentioned for PSG, the SIT provides an interesting and probably less expensive test to confirm a clinical diagnosis. It also remains to be answered to what extent this test can be used for the assessment of severity and treatment response. At present large-scale studies are being performed that might help to evaluate whether the SIT is a reliable tool to assess treatment response.

ACTIGRAPHY

Because of the pronounced day-to-day variability of RLS symptoms in many patients, it seems advisable to develop ambulatory diagnostic instruments that can provide information on the severity of symptoms over extended periods of time. This combined with the need to reduce the costs of health care, has led to the development of portable devices that can be used for ambulatory assessment. Although PSG still remains the most widely used diagnostic tool, actimetry is generally accepted as a promising and useful device for research and diagnostic screening. Actimetry employs a small portable device capable of sensing physical motion and storing the resulting information (Figure 9.15). It is widely used to evaluate rest–activity cycles in the healthy population, as well as in sleep disorders such as insomnia, circadian-rhythm disorders and RLS. Modern actigraphs have a movement detector and sufficient memory to record for long periods of time. They can be taken outside the sleep laboratory be self-applied, and may even be transmitted by e-mail[12].

The use of actigraphy in sleep disorders such as restless legs syndrome (RLS) with periodic limb movements (PLM) has gained popularity over recent years. These devices, called actimeters, are used to record limb movements (wrist or ankle). When applied to the ankle (Figure 9.16), the actimeter can record periodic leg movements over the entire recording period, sometimes over a week. Thus, PLMs are recorded and quantified regardless of whether the patient is awake or asleep[20]. The data collected are displayed on a computer and are examined for activity versus inactivity, and hence analyzed for wake versus sleep. The actimetric monitor detects motor activity in any direction, stores the data in its memory and, when downloaded by

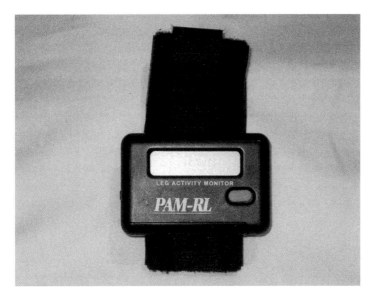

Figure 9.15 Actimeter

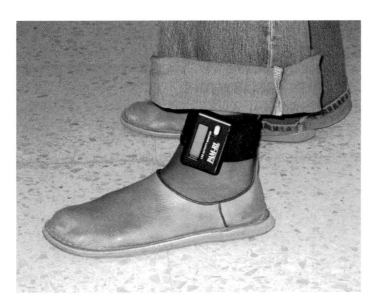

Figure 9.16 Portable ankle actimetry device

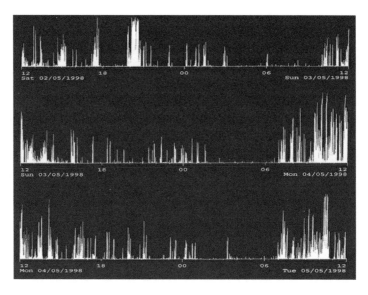

Figure 9.17 *Actigraphic recording in restless legs syndrome*

means of an interface, transmits the results to a computer for analysis. The method of analysis is based on 'threshold crossing' or 'reference level comparison', basing measurements on the frequency of activity (with respect to the time domain) to evaluate the rest/activity cycle, respectively[12]. The results of actimetry improved if combined with information provided by a sleep diary. Several studies observed that it correlates well with the results obtained during PSG in a sleep laboratory. Thus Kazenwadel and associates[20] found a high correlation between actimetry and anterior tibialis muscle surface EMG for the PLM index. One of the more intuitive uses of the ambulatory activity monitoring is to assess PLMs that occur both during sleep and waking (PLMS and PLMW) (Figure 9.17).

Actimetry has been used in two double-blind studies on treatment efficacy[21,22]. Its use over several nights was helpful to confirm the stability of therapeutic effects.

The advantages of actimetry are its simplicity, its ability to record for long time periods (from minutes to several days), its low-cost monitoring in all environments (excluding water), its ability to be used in a home environment minimizing typical 'laboratory effects' that may alter a patient's typical sleep patterns, and its reliability in all kind of patients (including demented patients and those not compliant with PSG, such as small children)[11,12]. Furthermore, actimetry may provide an opportunity for subjects to adhere more closely than PSG to their usually scheduled bedtime and wake-up time, thus providing a more accurate estimate of typical sleep duration than PSG does. Moreover, it may be useful for epidemiological studies in selected populations or to study motor habits during sleep[23].

However, actimetry also has some limitations[24,25] in patients with RLS and PLM: it is limited by its tendency to underestimate the frequency of leg movements during sleep, and it does not provide information on sleep stages. Furthermore, it does not help to categorize the pattern or intensity of movements, and is thus not valid to evaluate specific movement disorders. Overall, actimetry performs best at estimating total sleep time (i.e. normal subjects). However, when sleep is fragmented (i.e. in RLS with high PLM index and an increase in awakenings), it becomes less accurate for the detection of sleep and waking, overestimating sleep and underestimating waking, particularly during the day when an individual is more likely to sit quietly while awake. Furthermore, as there is no accurate marker of bedtime, the determination of sleep latency or variables whose calculations depend on it (sleep efficiency and wake after sleep onset) become unreliable.

The clinical value of actimetry

Actimetry is a specific technique for the quantification and recording of movements and for the study of conditions associated to physiologic or peculiar motor patterns[12]. Norms need to be established and standardized before actimetry can be used with full confidence in sleep/wake studies. This process of standardization needs to take place before its use can become widespread, and would be similar to that developed for PSG in 1968 by Rechtshaffen and Kales[24,26].

Although actimetry is still not routinely used in the diagnosis of RLS, it is a useful tool in the assessment of treatment efficacy[12,21,24].

Activity monitoring can discriminate between actual movements and EMG potentials occurring without any significant displacement of a limb, even though it provides relatively unspecific results[12].

The main function of actimetry is the measurement of night-to-night changes in sleep patterns of an individual, a function that is of great value for the assessment of treatment effects and other factors that affect the consistency of a patient's sleep[24].

Actimetry represents a less expensive approach than PSG and has the added benefit of being able to record over longer periods of time. It is particularly useful for the evaluation of circadian rhythm disorders (i.e. delayed or advanced sleep phase syndrome and shift work), as it provides information that frequently would not be obtainable in any other practical way[24].

Actimetry is useful in the evaluation of sleep in individuals that might not tolerate PSG, such as children and demented elderly[11,12,24].

CONCLUSIONS

Sleep laboratory methods, although not strictly necessary for the diagnosis of RLS, offer an interesting alternative to support the diagnosis of RLS objectively. The best known instrumental diagnostic test is polysomnography (PSG). However, because of its cost, newer, less-expensive alternatives have been developed, such as the Suggested Immobilization Test (SIT) or actimetry. Some of these tests offer the advantage of being suitable for the home environment, and can record information over longer periods of time. Their wider use might be helpful not only for research purposes, but also for the assessment of severity and treatment response in the clinical setting.

REFERENCES

1. Walters AS. Toward a better definition of the restless legs syndrome. The International Restless Legs Syndrome Study Group. *Mov Disord* 1995;10: 634–42

2. Allen RP, Picchietti D, Hening WA, *et al*. Restless legs syndrome: diagnostic criteria, special considerations, and epidemiology. A report from the restless legs syndrome diagnosis and epidemiology workshop at the National Institutes of Health. *Sleep Med* 2003;4:101–19

3. Thorpy M, Ehrenberg BL, Hening WA, *et al*. Restless legs syndrome – detection and management in primary care. *Am Fam Physician* 2000;62:108–14

4. Allen RP, Earley CJ. Restless legs syndrome: a review of clinical and pathophysiologic features. *J Clin Neurophysiol* 2001;18:128–47

5. Montplaisir J, Boucher S, Poirier G, *et al*. Clinical, polysomnographic, and genetic characteristics of restless legs syndrome: a study of 133 patients diagnosed with new standard criteria. *Mov Disord* 1997;12:61–5

6. Trenkwalder C. *Restless Legs Syndrome: Klinik, Differentialdiagnose, Neurophysiologie; Therapie*. Berlin, Heidelberg, New York: Springer, 1998

7. Winkelmann J, Wetter TC, Collado-Seidel V, *et al*. Clinical characteristics and frequency of the hereditary restless legs syndrome in a population of 300 patients. *Sleep* 2000;23:597–602

8. Michaud M, Paquet J, Lavigne G, *et al*. Sleep laboratory diagnosis of restless legs syndrome. *Eur Neurol* 2002;48:108–13

9. Montplaisir J, Boucher S, Nicolas A, *et al*. Immobilization tests and periodic leg movements in sleep for the diagnosis of restless leg syndrome. *Mov Disord* 1998;13:324–9

10. Allen RP, Earley CJ. Validation of the Johns Hopkins Restless Legs Severity Scale. *Sleep Med* 2001;3:239–42

11. Chervin RD. Use of clinical tools and test in sleep medicine. In Kryger M, Roth T, Dement W, (eds). *Principles and Practice of Sleep Medicine*, 3rd edn. Philadelphia: WB Saunders, 2000:538

12. Malow BA, Aldrich MS. Polysomnography. In Chokroverty S, Hening WA, Walters AS, (eds). *Sleep and Movements Disorders*, 1st edn. Philadelphia: Butterworth-Heinemann, 2003:125–31

13. Hornyak M, Kotterba S, Trenkwalder C, and Members of the Study Group 'Motor Disorders' of the German Sleep Society. Indication for performing polysomnography in the diagnosis and treatment of restless legs syndrome. *Somnologie* 2001;5:159–62

14. Brodeur C, Montplaisir J, Godbout R, *et al*. Treatment of restless legs syndrome and periodic leg movements during sleep with L-dopa: a double-blind, controlled study. *Neurology* 1988;1845–8

15. Nicolas A, Michaud M, Lavigne G, *et al*. The influence of sex, age and sleep/wake state on characteristics of periodic leg movements in restless legs syndrome patients. *Clin Neurophysiol* 1999;110:1168–74

16. Pelletier G, Lorrain D, Montplaisir J. Sensory and motor components of the restless legs syndrome. *Neurology* 1992;42:1663–6

17. Coleman RM, Pollak CP, Weitzman ED. Periodic movements in sleep (nocturnal myoclonus): relation to sleep disorders. *Ann Neurol* 1980;8:416–21

18. Karadeniz D, Ondze B, Besset A, *et al*. Are periodic leg movements during sleep (PLMS) responsible for sleep disruption in insomnia patients? *Eur J Neurol* 2000;7:331–6

19. Michaud M, Lavigne G, Desautels A, *et al*. Effects of immobility on sensory and motor symptoms of restless legs syndrome. *Mov Disord* 2002;17:112–15

20. Kazenwadel J, Pollmacher T, Trenkwalder C, *et al*. New actigraphic assessment method for periodic leg movements (PLM). *Sleep* 1995;18:689–97

21. Trenkwalder C, Stiasny K, Pollmacher T, *et al*. L-dopa therapy of uremic and idiopathic restless legs syndrome: a double-blind, crossover trial. *Sleep* 1995; 18:681–8

22. Collado-Seidel V, Kazenwadel J, Wetter TC, *et al*. A controlled study of additional sr-L-dopa in L-dopa-responsive restless legs syndrome with late-night symptoms. *Neurology* 1999;52:285–90

23. Reyner LA, Horne JA, Reyner A. Gender- and age-related differences in sleep determined by home-recorded sleep logs and actimetry from 400 adults. *Sleep* 1995;18:127–34

24. Ancoli-Israel S, Cole R, Alessi C, *et al*. The role of actigraphy in the study of sleep and circadian rhythms. *Sleep* 2003;26:342–92

25. Ancoli-Israel S, Kripke DF, Klauber MR, *et al*. Periodic limb movements in sleep community dwelling elderly. *Sleep* 1991;14:496–500

26. Rechtschaffen A, Kales A (eds). *A Manual of Standardized Terminology: Techniques and Scoring System for Sleep Stages of Human Subjects*. Los Angeles, California: UCLA Brain Information Service/Brain Research Institute, 1968

10   Summary and conclusions

K. Ray Chaudhuri

As discussed in the preceding chapters, restless legs syndrome (RLS) is a common condition – and is the commonest movement disorder known. In spite of its widespread occurrence and its accepted morbidity, the condition continues to be largely under-recognized within medical communities and, as such, treatment remains far from ideal, although very effective treatment strategies are available. Part of this problem may arise from the fact that RLS is not a fatal disorder and its symptoms, usually paroxysmal, if not analyzed properly may suggest a psychological morbidity. There is also a commonly mistaken perception that RLS only occurs during sleep, whereas in reality, the symptoms also occur during quiet wakefulness and during daytime.

There is increasing research and awareness of the impact of RLS on activities of daily living, and publications are more robust since the International Restless Legs Syndrome Study Group (IRLSSG) defined diagnostic criteria in 1995. There is also increasing media coverage of RLS in both the USA and Europe. However, in many Western countries, RLS still remains a condition of low priority even if the patients may feel neglected, poorly treated and sometimes driven to depression because of chronic sleeplessness.

In the USA, there are prominent patient groups serving the interests of RLS patients (see Contact points). In the UK, until 2001, the Ekbom Support Group, led by Mrs E. Gill, was the only patient support group. In 2001, RLS:UK, a multidisciplinary academic-led group was formed to develop awareness and research into RLS in the UK. With the support of the Ekbom Support Group in the UK, Dr L. Appiah-Kubi from the Restless Legs Syndrome Group of the UK (RLS:UK) analyzed the results of questionnaires sent out to some RLS sufferers in the UK registered with the Ekbom Support Group. Among 400 questionnaires returned, a minority had seen a neurologist for RLS and a majority had tried herbal treatment or vitamin supplementation as treatment for RLS by themselves. Among those who saw their general practitioners, most were prescribed benzodiazepines, analgesia, antidepressants and quinine in descending order, in spite of availability of effective treatment strategies with dopamine agonists.

A minority were prescribed levodopa and even less dopamine agonists. In this series, 28% were never seen by any physicians and only 13% were taking dopaminergic treatment which is generally thought to be first line therapy for RLS. In clinical practice in the UK, it is common to see patients who may have had the condition for 10 or more years before the diagnosis is made. Although ascertainment bias is a problem with such questionnaire studies, this survey indicated that RLS in the UK remains under-recognized and largely inappropriately treated. This observation may be true for most European countries and parts of the USA (R.P. Allen, Personal Communication).

In the white Caucasian population, adult prevalence figures of RLS range between 5% and 29% although, based on more robust studies, a range of 7–10% appears to be more probable.

Recent data from the questionnaire-based REST study (RLS epidemiology, symptoms and treatment), which targeted the primary care and general population in five European countries and the US, suggested a prevalence figure of 8.6% for RLS in the UK with 3.9% of this population suffering from moderate-to-very severe symptoms. In the general population survey, disturbed or poor-quality sleep was the most common troublesome symptom reported followed by pain and inability to get comfortable. Only 1.2% of those in primary care and 6.7% in the general population had received a diagnosis of RLS. This survey also showed a considerable impact of RLS on quality of life as measured by the SF-36 scale.

Although the diagnosis is often made in middle age, on enquiry, symptoms often date back to childhood. Historically there may be a link to childhood 'growing pains' or 'hyperactivity'. It is interesting to note that the MEMO study[1], a population-based survey of an elderly population, reported an overall prevalence of 9.8% and a higher prevalence of RLS with advancing age in women. It was noteworthy that RLS patients reported a higher incidence of depression ($p = 0.012$) and lower self-reported mental health scores ($p = 0.029$) than did non-RLS cases. There was a considerable impact on self-perceived mental health, and quality of life as measured by scales such as the SF36. Currently, little data are available in relation to the prevalence of RLS in other ethnic groups such as Asian or Black populations, although observations in Singapore and Northern India (Delhi) suggest that RLS may be relatively uncommon in Asian subjects (see Chapter 3). Epidemiological reports of RLS in African or African-Caribbean populations are not available. Prevalence figures for RLS in the UK are not currently available but, extrapolating from the MEMO study, there are likely to be in excess of five million people with RLS in the UK. Many will have a mild form of RLS, but in some the symptoms may be very severe and these patients will often request and need treatment.

Although the cause of primary RLS is unknown, there is a strong link with iron metabolism and also with dopamine levels in the brain, particularly the striatal region. However, the relation is not a simple one; in the MEMO study, no evidence was found that iron or ferritin deficiency was a major cause of RLS, although there were only a small number of RLS cases. These issues have been discussed in Chapter 6 by W. Ondo. The genetic basis of RLS has been elucidated more recently with description of linkage of families to chromosome 12q and 14q, although no gene has yet been found. Much work is now under way to find a gene or genes responsible for the symptoms of RLS. Work from Allen and co-workers suggests that the phenotype of RLS may depend upon the age at onset of symptoms with those presenting before the age of 40–50 years haveing a strong familial pattern[2].

It is worth noting that the diagnosis of RLS is essentially clinical and is made by taking a good and thorough clinical history from the subject and partner. RLS should not be confused with painful conditions of the legs such as arthritis of hip or knee and positional discomfort. All cases should have iron deficiency anemia excluded and in selected cases screening for neuropathy may be required. Serum levels of ferritin (the primary storage unit for iron and known to correlate inversely with RLS severity) should be checked.

The three main partially reversible causes of RLS are:
- Pregnancy
- Renal disease
- Iron deficiency anemia

Reassuringly however, inspite of the uncertainties about the pathophysiologic basis of RLS, dopaminergic treatments and dopamine agonists may offer sustained benefit and in some cases dramatic reversal in deterioration of quality of life. Not all patients, however, require treatment. In some, lifestyle changes may be useful. These include dietary supplementation with iron if iron deficiency anemia is demonstrated (particularly if ferritin levels fall below 50 ng/ml), mineral supplements (magnesium, potassium and calcium) and good sleep hygiene. Thus knowledge of RLS needs to disseminated more vigorously to the medical communities to ensure appropriate and timely treatment. Some drugs may worsen RLS – these include antidepressants, calcium antagonists, anti-hypertensive agents, anti-nausea medications (except domperidone), phenytoin, some anti-histamines, tranquilizers and high intake of caffeine.

As indicated above, RLS is the commonest movement disorder known and affects sleep as well as daytime function. The exact impact of chronic RLS on daytime functions such as work and driving remains unclear because of lack of data. In the UK, RLS continues to be regarded as a psychosomatic disorder and patients are often told 'to put up with it' in spite of availability of very effective treatment strategies. In practice, it is not unusual to see RLS patients whose diagnosis has been delayed by years, and lack of appropriate treatment has rendered the patient severely sleep deprived and depressed, even to the point of suicide. It is time therefore, to reverse the notion that RLS is 'the commonest disorders you have never heard of'.

CONTACT POINTS

UK

Eileen Gill at the Ekbom Support Group keeps a list of specialists with an interest in the management of RLS. In the UK, information in relation to RLS may also be obtained from the newly formed RLS:UK group, a multi-disciplinary group aiming to advance knowledge and understanding of RLS in the UK. Contact points are through Eileen Gill (gill@ekbom-88.demon.co.uk).

Australia
Beverly Yakich
15 Carpenter Crescent
Warriewood
NSW 2102
Australia
nicc@mail.com
www.rls.org.au

Austria
Birgit E. Hogl MD
Department of Neurology
Universitätskliniken Innsbruck
Anichstr. 35
6020 Innsbruck
Austria
birgit.ho@uibk.ac.at

Waltraud Moldaschl
Puchheimgasse 5
3860 Heidenreichstein
Austria
w.moldaschl@gmx.at
www.restless-legs.at

Denmark
Stig Eric Weibel
Hornbaekvej 666 b
Hornbaek Sjaelland 3100
Denmark
restless@legs.dk

Finland
Markku Partinen MD, PhD
University of Helsinki
Makipellontie 15
00320 Helsinki
Finland
markku.partinen@rinnekoti.fi
www.uniliitto.fi

France
Guy Bourhis MD
France
bourhis@lasc.univ-metz.fr

Germany
Wolfgang Berger
Schwarz BioSciences
Alfred-Nobel-Strasse 10
40789 Monheim am Rhein
Germany
wolfgang.berger@schwarzbio-sciences.com

Karin Stiasny-Kolster MD
Department of Neurology
Phillips Universität Marburg
Rudolf-Bultmann-Strasse 8
35039 Marburg
Germany
stiasny@staff.uni-marburg.de

Greece

Georgios M. Hadjigeorgiou MD
Department of Neurology
University of Thessaly
Medical School
23rd Oktobriou 15
41222 Larissa
Greece
gmhadji@med.uth.gr

Italy

Luigi Ferini-Strambi MD
Department of Neurology
San Raffaele
Via Stamira d'Ancona 20
20127 Milan
Italy
ferinistrambi.luigi@hsz.it

Marco Zucconi MD
Department of Neurology
San Raffaele Scientific Institute
  and Hospital
Via Stamira d'Ancona 20
20129 Milan
Italy
zucconi.marco@hsr.it

The Netherlands

Joke Jaarsma
Quinten Massijsstraat 5-II
1077 MC Amsterdam
The Netherlands
j.jaarsma@planet.nl
www.stichting-restless-legs.org

New Zealand

Moira Robinson
2 Trinity Lane
Richmond Nelson 7002
New Zealand
mcrobinson@xtra.co.nz

Spain

Renata Egatz MD
Sleep Disorder Unit
Department of Neurology
Fundación Jiménez Díaz
Avda Reyes Católicos 2
28040 Madrid
Spain
regatz@fjd.es

Diego Garcia-Borreguero MD
Sleep Disorder Unit
Department of Neurology
Avda Reyes Católicos 2
28040 Madrid
Spain
dgarciaborreguero@fjd.es

Sweden

Gunnel Stahl
Skulptorvagen 16
12143 Johanneshov
Sweden
stahl.gunnel@telia.com
www.restlesslegs.nu

Switzerland

Claudio Bassetti
Neurology Department
University Hospital of Zurich
Frauenklinikstr. 26
8091 Zurich
Switzerland
claudio.bassetti@usz.ch

Turkey

Derya Kaynak MD
University of Istanbul
Department of Neurology
Sleep Disorders Unit
Cerrahpasa Medical School
University of Istanbul
Istanbul 34303
Turkey
kaynak@attglobal.net

UK

Eileen Gill
18 Rodbridge Drive
Thorpe Bay
Southend-on-Sea
Essex SS1 3DF
UK
gill@ekbom-88.demon.co.uk
www.restlesslegs.org.uk

Frauke Stegie
Research Nurse
Dayhospital
University Hospital Lewisham
Lewisham High Street
London, SE13 6 LH
UK
franke.stegie@uhl.nhs.uk

USA

Georgianna Bell
RLS Foundation
819 Second Street SW
Rochester
MN 55902,
USA
bell@rls.org
www.rls.org

Allan O'Bryan
RLS Foundation
819 Second Street SW
Rochester MN 55902
USA
obryan@rls.org
www.rls.org

Web sites

www.restlesslegs.org.uk
   www.welcome.to/ekbom
   http://www.wemove.org/rls_mdc.html
   http://www.rls.org/

REFERENCES

1.   Rothdach AJ, Trenkwalder C, Haberstock J, *et al*. Prevalence and risk factors of RLS in an elderly population. The MEMO study. *Neurology* 2000;54:1064–8

2.   Allen RP, La Buda MC, Becker P, et al. Family history study of restless legs syndrome. *Sleep Med* 2002;3:53–7

Index

Page numbers of tables and illustrations are in italic